ADA **Dental Drug** Handbook:
A Quick Reference

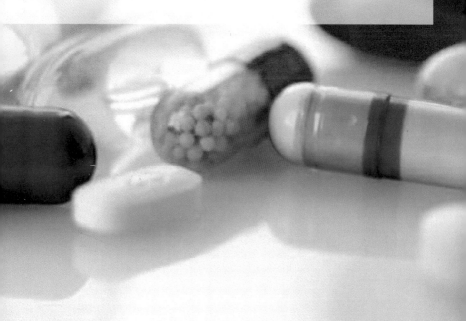

ADA **American Dental Association**®

America's leading advocate for oral health

Acknowledgements

The American Dental Association's Science Institute and the Department of Product Development and Sales developed this publication following a request by the ADA New Dentist Committee in 2015.

Principal contributions to this manuscript were made by Jay Elkareh, Pharm.D., Ph.D, Manager, Product Evaluation, Science Institute; Anita Mark, Senior Scientific Content Specialist, ADA Science Institute; Kathy Pulkrabek, Manager/Editor, Professional Products, Department of Product Development and Sales; and Carolyn Tatar, MBA, Senior Manager, Product Development and Sales at the American Dental Association.

External contributions to this manuscript were made by The ADA Dental Drug Handbook Editorial Advisory Panel: Sebastian Ciancio, DDS, MS, Director, Center for Clinical Dental Studies, and Adjunct Professor of Pharmacology, University at Buffalo School of Dental Medicine; Paul Eleazer, DDS, MS, Professor and Chair, Department of Endodontics, University of Alabama School of Dentistry; and Paul A. Moore, DMD, PhD, MPH, Professor, Pharmacology, Dental Anesthesiology and Dental Public Health, University of Pittsburgh School of Dental Medicine.

This book was designed by Lisa Empleo of Gray Cat Graphic Design.

The American Dental Association (ADA), the authors and editors (together the "Publishers") publish and present the ADA Dental Drug Handbook to you. This handbook does not constitute policy of the ADA, establish a standard of care or restrict a dentist's exercise of professional judgment. As the science of dental therapeutics evolves, changes in drug treatment and use become necessary. The reader is advised to consult the package insert for each drug to consider and adopt all safety precautions, before use, particularly with new and infrequently used drugs. The reader is responsible for ascertaining the U.S. Food and Drug Administration clearance of each drug and device used in his or her practice. Many of the proprietary names of the products listed in this book are trademarked and registered in the U.S. Patent Office. It should be understood that by making this material available, the Publishers are not advocating the use of any product described herein, nor are the Publishers responsible for misuse of a product due to typographical error. Additional information on any product may be obtained from the manufacturer.

Most of the chapters in the handbook will include drug monographs. These monographs give a broad pharmacological overview of the many drugs used in dentistry (e.g., drug interactions, adverse drug reactions, pharmacokinetics, contraindications, etc.). The clinical information has been compiled from various sources such as the U.S. Food & Drug Administration (*www.fda.gov*), Epocrates (*www. epocrates.com*), Lexicomp (*online.lexi.com*), Medscape (*www.medscape.com*). For a comprehensive drug profile, please refer to the previously mentioned websites or see the drug package insert.

Most of the monographs include a sample prescription. Clinicians are responsible to adjust the prescription dose, frequency and length of treatment based on the procedure performed, the medicine prescribed, and the patient condition, such as age, weight, metabolism, liver and renal function. The sample prescription in the handbook represents only a general recommendation by the authors based on scientific literature, and expert insights.

The Publishers have produced this handbook in their individual capacities and not on behalf or in the interest of any pharmaceutical companies or state or federal agencies. This handbook does not provide legal advice, and readers must consult with their own attorneys for such advice. The Publishers disclaim all responsibility for any liability, loss, injury or damage resulting directly or indirectly from the reader's use and application of the information in this book and make no representations or warranties with respect to such information, including the products described herein.

Table of Contents

Contributors

Erica Brecher, DMD, MS
Assistant Professor, Department of Pediatric
  Dentistry
Virginia Commonwealth University School
  of Dentistry
Richmond, Virginia

Elias Mikael Chatah, DMD, B. Pharm, MS
Assistant Clinical Professor
Group Practice Leader
University of Connecticut School of Dental
  Medicine
Farmington, Connecticut

Sebastian Ciancio, DDS, MS
Distinguished Service Professor and Chair
Department of Periodontics & Endodontics
Adjunct Professor of Pharmacology
Director, Center for Clinical Dental Studies
University at Buffalo School of Dental Medicine
Buffalo, New York

Paul Eleazer, DDS, MS
Professor and Chair, Department of Endodontics
University of Alabama School of Dentistry
Birmingham, Alabama

Jay Elkareh, PharmD, PhD
Manager, Product Evaluation
Science Institute
American Dental Association
Chicago, Illinois

Louis Erazo, BS
Clinical Research Associate, Acceptance Program
Science Institute
American Dental Association
Chicago, Illinois

Elliot V. Hersh, DMD, MS, PhD
Professor, Oral Surgery and Pharmacology
Director, Division of Pharmacology and
  Clinical Therapeutics
University of Pennsylvania School of
  Dental Medicine
Philadelphia, Pennsylvania

Martha Ann Keels, DDS, PhD
Adjunct Professor in Pediatric Dentistry
University of North Carolina School of Dentistry
Associate Consulting Associate Professor
  in Surgery
Adjunct Associate Professor in Pediatrics
Duke University
Private Practice, Pediatric Dentistry
Durham, North Carolina

Paul A. Moore, DMD, PhD, MPH
Professor, Pharmacology, Dental
Anesthesiology and Dental Public Health
University of Pittsburgh School of Dental
Medicine
Pittsburgh, Pennsylvania

Lida Radfar, DDS, MS
Diplomat, American Board of Oral Medicine
Clinical Professor of Oral Medicine, Oral
Diagnosis and Radiology Department
University of Oklahoma College of Dentistry
Oklahoma City, Oklahoma

S. Craig Rhodes, DMD, MSD
Associate Professor and Director, Graduate
Endodontics
Center for Advanced Dental Education
Saint Louis University
St. Louis, Missouri

**Lakshmanan Suresh, DDS, MS, PhD,
D(ABMLI), D(ABOMP)**
Clinical Professor, Department of Oral
  Diagnostic Sciences
School of Dental Medicine
State University of New York at Buffalo
Buffalo, New York

Kathleen M. Ziegler, PharmD
Manager, Scientific Information
Science Institute
American Dental Association
Chicago, Illinois

Preface

This ADA handbook is designed to serve not only as a clinical educational resource but also to promote clinical best practices to all dental professionals. The handbook presents a range of information in a concise, attractive, easy-to-follow format. It is intended for use by practicing dentists, students, dental educators and the entire dental team to assist them in the treatment of patients. The goal was to create an indispensable, "go to" drug reference for dental professionals.

Patients are being prescribed more medications today than ever before. Due in part to our aging and mobile population, dentists are confronted with many considerations when treating patients. Patients seeking dental care are often using a wide range of medications for various medical problems. In addition, both dentist and patient have many choices to make about the variety of products available today for treating disorders of the mouth.

In ADA-sponsored focus groups, practicing dentists have expressed a need for a quick and accurate drug reference developed specifically for them. This handbook is based on what those dentists told us they need to make their practices complete: concise and accurate information about the medications they use. They wanted information that was based on the best practices of science and pharmacology and organized by drug category.

The book contains five sections; the main section focuses on drugs used by the dentist. Each chapter starts with a brief overview of the category and contains easy-to-use drug monographs with sample prescriptions, contraindications, precautions, drug interactions, common side effects and more. Other sections include pediatric management, dental office emergencies, handling patients with specific medical conditions and useful tables.

A team of dentists, pharmacists, scientists, and experts in pharmacology have worked together to create a unique, complete, and easy-to-read therapeutics publication for dental profession and beyond.

Jay Elkareh, Pharm.D., Ph.D.
Editor
Manager, Product Evaluation
Science Institute
American Dental Association

Drugs Used in **Dentistry**

Chapter 1:
Analgesics and Acute Pain Management

Kathleen Ziegler, PharmD

Overview

Pain management is an integral part of dental practice. There are two main types of pain: nociceptive, which is treated with nonopioid and opioid analgesics; or neuropathic, which is treated with adjunctive agents such as anticonvulsant and antidepressant medications. This chapter will focus on oral nonopioid and opioid analgesics. These conventional analgesics either interrupt ascending nociceptive impulses or depress their communication within the central nervous system.

Depending on the dental intervention performed, acute postprocedural pain can be anticipated to be mild, moderate, or severe (Table 1).

In 2016, the ADA House of Delegates adopted a statement on the use of opioids in the treatment of dental pain, which stated, "Dentists should consider nonsteroidal anti-inflammatory analgesics as the first-line therapy for acute pain management."

Table 1. Anticipated postprocedural pain according to dental intervention	
Intervention	**Anticipated Postprocedural Pain**
Frenectomy Gingivectomy Routine endodontics Scaling/root planing Simple extraction Subgingival restorative procedures	Mild
Implant surgery Quadrant periodontal flap surgery with bony recontouring Surgical endodontics Surgical extraction	Moderate
Complex implant Partial or full bony impaction surgery Periodontal surgery	Severe

1 | Strategy for Dental Pain Management

If pain is anticipated to last 24 to 48 hours following the procedure, patients are advised to take the prescribed medication on a regularly scheduled basis for the 1st two days to prevent pain recurrence when plasma drug levels fall off between doses. The remainder of the medication can be taken "as needed" (i.e., prn) for breakthrough pain.

One algorithm for management of various levels of dental pain was developed by Moore and Hersh. Using the anticipated pain level following a dental procedure, they recommended a stepwise management plan (Table 2).

Other therapeutic strategies include administration of NSAIDs 1 hour prior to the procedure and use of longer-acting local anesthetics (e.g., bupivacaine 0.5% with 1:200,000 epinephrine) during the immediate postoperative period. Also, perioperative administration of a corticosteroid (e.g., dexamethasone) may limit inflammation and decrease pain following third-molar extractions (See Chapter 8: Oral Lesions and Corticosteroids).

Table 2. Analgesic Use According to Pain Level	
Anticipated Pain Level	**Analgesic Recommendation**
Mild	Single-agent ibuprofen 200 to 400 mg as needed for pain every 4 to 6 hours
Mild to Moderate	Single-agent ibuprofen 400 to 600 mg fixed interval every 6 hours for 24 hours *then* Single-agent ibuprofen 400 mg as needed for pain every 4 to 6 hours
Moderate to Severe	Ibuprofen 400 to 600 mg plus acetaminophen 500 mg fixed interval every 6 hours for 24 hours *then* Ibuprofen 400 mg plus acetaminophen 500 mg as needed for pain every 6 hours
Severe	Ibuprofen 400 to 600 mg plus acetaminophen 650 mg with hydrocodone 10 mg fixed interval every 6 hours for 24 to 48 hours *then* Ibuprofen 400 to 600 mg plus acetaminophen 500 mg as needed for pain every 6 hours

Adapted from: Moore PA, Hersh EV. Combining ibuprofen and acetaminophen for acute pain management after third-molar extractions: translating clinical research to dental practice. J Am Dent Assoc 2013;144(8):898-908.

2 | Nonopioid Analgesics

The nonopioid analgesics include acetaminophen, aspirin and other NSAIDs. The maximum analgesic effect of acetaminophen or aspirin usually occurs with single doses between 650 and 1300 mg. For NSAIDs other than aspirin, the analgesic ceiling may be somewhat higher. One advantage is that tolerance does not develop to the analgesic effects of these drugs.

The anti-inflammatory and analgesic properties of NSAIDs, as well as most of their adverse effects, result from their inhibition of cyclooxygenase (COX), which is a key enzyme in the production of postoperative pain and inflammation due to its ability to convert arachidonic acid to prostaglandins. Prostaglandins are mediators of inflammation, fever, and pain. Aspirin inactivates COX by irreversible acetylation, whereas the newer NSAIDs are reversible competitive inhibitors of COX. Most NSAIDs bind weakly and reversibly to platelet COX, interfering with platelet aggregation only until the drug is cleared from the system; however, because aspirin irreversibly binds platelet COX, platelet function is permanently affected for the life of the platelet (8 to 10 days). Prostaglandins also have a role in GI mucosal protection and play an essential role in renal perfusion; this accounts for the potential of NSAIDs to cause gastrointestinal complications (i.e., bleeding) and nephrotoxicity, respectively.

The mechanism of action of acetaminophen is less clear compared with NSAIDs; however, it is thought to involve inhibition of prostaglandin synthesis within the central nervous system.

3 | Opioid Analgesics

Opioid analgesics can be categorized as full agonists, partial agonists, or mixed agonist/antagonists. Full agonists are generally used for treatment of moderate-to-severe acute or chronic pain. Unlike NSAIDs, most opioids have no ceiling for their analgesic effectiveness, except that imposed by development of adverse effects.

The precise mechanism of the analgesic action of opioids is unknown. However, specific central nervous system opioid receptors for endogenous compounds with opioid-like activity have been identified throughout the brain and spinal cord and are thought to play a role in the analgesic effects of these drugs.

Risks of these drugs include nausea and vomiting, drowsiness, respiratory depression, potential addiction, abuse, and misuse.

📖 | Suggested Reading List

- American Dental Association. Statement on the Use of Opioids in the Treatment of Dental Pain. 2016. *https://www.ada.org/en/press-room/news-releases/2018-archives/february/american-dental-association-statement-on-opioids.* Accessed August 3, 2018.
- Becker DE. Pain management: Part 1: Managing acute and postoperative dental pain. Anesth Prog 2010;57(2):67-78.
- Ganzberg S, Fricton J. Analgesics: Opioids and Nonopioids. In: ADA/PDR Guide to Dental Therapeutics, Ciancio SG, editor. 5th ed. Chicago: American Dental Association and Physician's Desk Reference, Inc., pp 63-133, 2009.
- Hersh EV, Kane WT, O'Neil MG, et al. Prescribing recommendations for the treatment of acute pain in dentistry. Compend Contin Educ Dent 2011;32(3):22, 24-30.

- Moore PA, Hersh EV. Combining ibuprofen and acetaminophen for acute pain management after third-molar extractions: translating clinical research to dental practice. J Am Dent Assoc 2013;144(8):898-908.
- Drugs for pain. Treat Guidel Med Lett 2013;11(128):31-42.

Drug Monograph

The following table lists some of the opioids and non-opioids analgesics commonly used in dentistry. The monographs below highlight a 4 days prescription, however, prescribers are encouraged to use their clinical judgment; the length of treatment might vary depending on the procedure performed and the patient's anticipated level of pain.

NOTE: The sample prescriptions in this handbook represent a general recommendation. Clinicians are responsible to adjust the prescription dose, frequency and length of treatment based on the procedure performed, the medicine prescribed, and the patient conditions such as age, weight, metabolism, liver and renal function.

Non-Opioids list:

Acetaminophen

Tablets: 325 mg, 500 mg, 650 mg · Chewable tablets: 80 mg, 160 mg
Liquid: 32 mg/mL, 100 mg/mL

ORAL CONDITIONS	· Dental pain management
SUGGESTED DIRECTIONS	· Take 2 tablets (2x 325 mg) every 6 hours for 4 days as needed (32 tablets) *maximum dose 4,000 mg/day* *manufacturers recommend 3,000 mg/day*

BLACK BOX WARNING – Hepatotoxicity: Acetaminophen has been associated with cases of acute liver failure, at times resulting in liver transplant and death especially at doses that exceed 4,000 mg per day, and often involving more than one acetaminophen-containing product.

CONTRAINDICATIONS	· Active and severe hepatic disease · Hypersensitivity to acetaminophen · Severe hepatic impairment
CAUTIONS	· Recent alcohol consumption increases risk of hepatic injury
MAJOR & SEVERE DRUG INTERACTIONS	· Concurrent use of acetaminophen and isoniazid may result in an increased risk of hepatotoxicity · Concurrent use of acetaminophen and imatinib may result in increased acetaminophen levels · Concurrent use of acetaminophen and warfarin may result in an increased risk of bleeding
ADVERSE DRUG REACTIONS	Common Reactions: · Pruritus · Constipation, nausea, vomiting · Headache, insomnia · Agitation · Atelectasis Less common reactions: · Generalized, acute exanthematous pustulosis, Stevens-Johnson syndrome, toxic epidermal necrolysis · Liver failure · Pneumonitis
PATIENT CONSIDERATIONS	· Pregnancy Category C · Lactation: amounts of acetaminophen secreted in milk are much less than doses usually given to infants · Elderly patients: no specific dosage adjustment is necessary · Renal failure: severe renal impairment (CrCl of 30 mL/min or less) increases risk of hepatic injury; dose reductions may be required · Hepatic disease: active hepatic disease or hepatic impairment increases risk of hepatic injury; dose reductions may be required · Recommend patient to keep hydrated and well-nourished while on medication to avoid hepatic injury
 **DRUG CONSIDERATIONS**	· Peak serum time: 0.5 to 1 hr · Half-life: 2 to 3 hours (adults) · Extensively metabolized in the liver · Excretion: less than 5% excreted unchanged in urine

Aspirin

Tablets: 81 mg, 325 mg, 500 mg, 650 mg

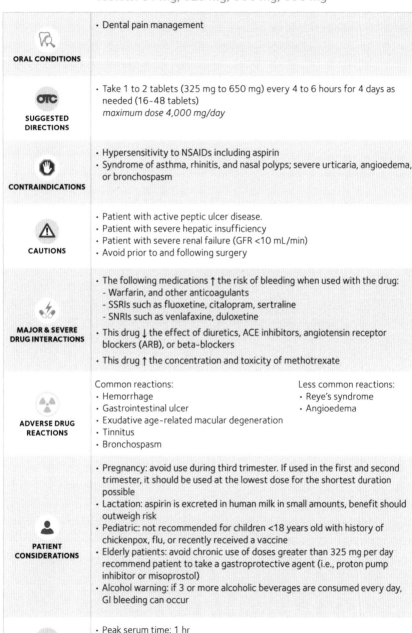

ORAL CONDITIONS	• Dental pain management
OTC **SUGGESTED DIRECTIONS**	• Take 1 to 2 tablets (325 mg to 650 mg) every 4 to 6 hours for 4 days as needed (16-48 tablets) *maximum dose 4,000 mg/day*
CONTRAINDICATIONS	• Hypersensitivity to NSAIDs including aspirin • Syndrome of asthma, rhinitis, and nasal polyps; severe urticaria, angioedema, or bronchospasm
CAUTIONS	• Patient with active peptic ulcer disease. • Patient with severe hepatic insufficiency • Patient with severe renal failure (GFR <10 mL/min) • Avoid prior to and following surgery

MAJOR & SEVERE DRUG INTERACTIONS	• The following medications ↑ the risk of bleeding when used with the drug:
	  - Warfarin, and other anticoagulants
	  - SSRIs such as fluoxetine, citalopram, sertraline
	  - SNRIs such as venlafaxine, duloxetine
	• This drug ↓ the effect of diuretics, ACE inhibitors, angiotensin receptor blockers (ARB), or beta-blockers
	• This drug ↑ the concentration and toxicity of methotrexate

ADVERSE DRUG REACTIONS	Common reactions: • Hemorrhage • Gastrointestinal ulcer • Exudative age-related macular degeneration • Tinnitus • Bronchospasm Less common reactions: • Reye's syndrome • Angioedema
PATIENT CONSIDERATIONS	• Pregnancy: avoid use during third trimester. If used in the first and second trimester, it should be used at the lowest dose for the shortest duration possible • Lactation: aspirin is excreted in human milk in small amounts, benefit should outweigh risk • Pediatric: not recommended for children <18 years old with history of chickenpox, flu, or recently received a vaccine • Elderly patients: avoid chronic use of doses greater than 325 mg per day recommend patient to take a gastroprotective agent (i.e., proton pump inhibitor or misoprostol) • Alcohol warning: if 3 or more alcoholic beverages are consumed every day, GI bleeding can occur
DRUG CONSIDERATIONS	• Peak serum time: 1 hr • Half-life: 20 to 60 minute • Excretion: >90% as metabolites in urine

Celecoxib
Tablets: 50 mg, 100 mg, 200 mg, 400 mg

ORAL CONDITIONS	• Chronic pain management
SAMPLE PRESCRIPTION	• Take 2 tablets (2x 200 mg) to start then 1 tablet (200 mg) every 12 hours for 4 days as needed (9 tablets)

BLACK BOX WARNING – Cardiovascular thrombotic events such as myocardial infarction and stroke. Gastrointestinal risk such as bleeding, ulceration, and perforation of the stomach or intestines.

CONTRAINDICATIONS	• Known hypersensitivity to celecoxib, or sulfonamides • History of asthma, urticaria, or major skin reactions after taking aspirin or other NSAIDs • Patient undergoing a coronary artery bypass graft (CABG) surgery
CAUTIONS	• Hepatotoxicity: discontinue if abnormal liver tests persist or worsen or if clinical signs and symptoms of liver disease develop. • Hypertension: monitor blood pressure • Heart failure and edema patients • Renal toxicity: monitor renal function in patients with renal impairment, heart failure, dehydration, or hypovolemia • Avoid use in pregnant women starting at 30 weeks of gestation • Hematologic toxicity: monitor hemoglobin or hematocrit in patients with any signs or symptoms of anemia

MAJOR & SEVERE DRUG INTERACTIONS	• This drug ↓ the effect of the following:
	  - Antihypertensive diuretics such as furosemide and thiazides
	  - Antihypertensive ACE inhibitors such as Lisinopril, and captopril
	  - Effect on platelets, including low dose aspirin
	• The following medications ↑ the adverse side effects of the drug:
	  - Anticoagulants and antiplatelet such as warfarin, and aspirin
	  - Antidepressant SSRIs such as fluoxetine, sertraline, citalopram
	  - Antiarrhythmic drugs such as digoxin

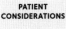 **ADVERSE DRUG REACTIONS**	Common reactions: • Abdominal pain, diarrhea, dyspepsia, flatulence • Peripheral edema, rash • Dizziness • Pharyngitis, Rhinitis, Sinusitis, Upper respiratory tract infection Less common reactions: • Hypertension • Headache • Insomnia
PATIENT CONSIDERATIONS	• Pregnancy Category C. Pregnancy Category D from 30 weeks of gestation onward (because of the risks of premature closure of the fetal ductus arteriosus) • Lactation: limited data, caution should be exercised • Pediatric: safety and effectiveness in patients younger than the age of 2 years have not been established • Elderly patients: start dosing at the low end of the dosing range, and monitor patients for adverse effects • Renal impairment: not recommended in patients with severe renal insufficiency • Hepatic impairment reduce dose by 50% in moderately impaired patients, and avoid in patients with severe hepatic impairment
DRUG CONSIDERATIONS	• Peak serum time: 3 hours • Highly protein bound • Half-life: 11 hours • Excretion: eliminated predominantly by hepatic metabolism with little (<3%) unchanged drug recovered in the urine and feces

Ibuprofen

Tablets: 100 mg, 200 mg · Chewable tablets: 50 mg, 100 mg
Tablets (Rx only): 400 mg, 600 mg, 800 mg · Liquid: 20 mg/mL, 40 mg/mL

ORAL CONDITIONS	· Dental pain management
SAMPLE PRESCRIPTION	· Take 1 tablet (600 mg) 3 to 4 times a day for 4 days as needed (12-16 tablets) *maximum 2,400 mg/day*
SUGGESTED DIRECTIONS	· Take 2 to 3 tablets (2x 200 mg to 3x 200 mg) 4 times a day for 4 days as needed (32-48 tablets) *maximum 2,400 mg/day*

BLACK BOX WARNING – Cardiovascular thrombotic events such as myocardial infarction and stroke. Gastrointestinal risk such as bleeding, ulceration, and perforation of the stomach or intestines.

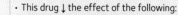 **CONTRAINDICATIONS**	· Hypersensitivity to NSAIDs including aspirin · Patients with history of peptic ulcer, or GI bleeding · Patient undergoing a coronary artery bypass graft (CABG) surgery.
CAUTIONS	· Patients with high blood pressure, heart disease · Patients with kidney disease, liver cirrhosis · Patients with uncontrolled diabetes, asthma, glaucoma · Patients with enlarged prostate, urinary incontinence

MAJOR & SEVERE DRUG INTERACTIONS	· This drug ↓ the effect of the following:
	  - Antihypertensive diuretics such as furosemide and thiazides
	  - Antihypertensive ACE inhibitors such as Lisinopril, and captopril
	  - Effect on platelets, including low dose aspirin
	· The following medications ↑ the adverse side effects of the drug:
	  - Anticoagulants and antiplatelet such as warfarin, and aspirin
	  - Antidepressant SSRIs such as fluoxetine, sertraline, citalopram

ADVERSE DRUG REACTIONS	Common reactions: · Epigastric pain, heartburn, nausea, vomiting, constipation, diarrhea · Skin rash · Dizziness, headache, tinnitus · Fluid retention Less common reactions: · Ocular adverse effects · Acute renal failure · Hypertension · Depression · Hematologic effects
PATIENT CONSIDERATIONS	· Pregnancy Category C; avoid during late pregnancy · Lactation: enters breast milk, compatible with breastfeeding · Pediatric: can be used in patients 6 months and older · Elderly patients: use with caution due to the higher risk of GI bleeding · Avoid in patients with advanced renal disease · No dose adjustments in patients with hepatic disease · Take with food, dairy products or products containing calcium
DRUG CONSIDERATIONS	· Peak serum time: 1 to 2 hours · More than 99% protein bound · Half-life: 1.8 to 2 hours · Little is excreted unchanged in urine

Naproxen

Tablets (OTC): 220 mg (Naproxen Sodium)
Tablets: 250 mg, 375 mg, 500 mg · Liquid: 25 mg/mL

ORAL CONDITIONS	• Dental pain management
SAMPLE PRESCRIPTION	• Take 1 tablet (500 mg) 2 times a day for 4 days as needed (8 tablets) *maximum 1,250 mg/day*
SUGGESTED DIRECTIONS	• Take 2 tablets (2x 220 mg) to start then 1 tablet (220 mg) every 8 to 12 hours for 4 days as needed (10-14 tablets) *maximum 3 tablets/day*

BLACK BOX WARNING – Cardiovascular thrombotic events such as myocardial infarction and stroke. Gastrointestinal risk such as bleeding, ulceration, and perforation of the stomach or intestines.

CONTRAINDICATIONS	• Hypersensitivity to NSAIDs or aspirin • Patients with history of peptic ulcer, or GI bleeding • Patient undergoing a coronary artery bypass graft (CABG) surgery
CAUTIONS	• Patients with high blood pressure, heart disease • Patients with kidney disease, liver cirrhosis • Patients with uncontrolled diabetes, asthma, glaucoma • Patients with enlarged prostate, urinary incontinence

MAJOR & SEVERE DRUG INTERACTIONS	• This drug ↓ the effect of the following:
	  - Antihypertensive diuretics such as furosemide and thiazides
	  - Antihypertensive ACE inhibitors such as Lisinopril, and captopril
	  - Effect on platelets, including low dose aspirin
	• The following medications ↑ the adverse side effects of the drug:
	  - Anticoagulants and antiplatelet such as warfarin, and aspirin
	  - Antidepressant SSRIs such as fluoxetine, sertraline, citalopram

ADVERSE DRUG REACTIONS	Common reactions: • Edema • Ecchymosis, pruritus, rash • Abdominal pain, constipation, heartburn, nausea • Dizziness, headache, somnolence • Ototoxicity, tinnitus • Dyspnea Less common reactions: • Angioedema • Acute renal failure • Hypertension • Bronchospasm • Hematologic effects
PATIENT CONSIDERATIONS	• Pregnancy Category C; avoid during late pregnancy • Lactation: enters breast milk, avoid if not necessary • Pediatric: safety and effectiveness in patients <2 years old has not been established • Elderly patients: use with caution and start at lower doses • Avoid in patients with moderate to advanced renal disease • Take with food, dairy products or products containing calcium
DRUG CONSIDERATIONS	• Bioavailability of naproxen is unaffected by food or time-of-day dosing • Peak serum time (naproxen sodium): 1 to 2 hours • Peak serum time (naproxen): 2 to 4 hours • Half-life: 12 to 17 hours • Excretion: approximately 95% of the naproxen from any dose is excreted in the urine, primarily as naproxen and metabolites

Opioids:

Opioids can be used as single agents or in combination with acetaminophen (APAP), aspirin (ASA), or ibuprofen. Codeine, dihydrocodeine, oxycodone, hyrocodone, hydromorphone, and tramadol.

Oxycodone's monograph is displayed below due to its common use as a single agent, while hyrocodone and codeine are rarely used as such. The properties of most opioids are somehow similar to that of oxycodone, and the monograph below can be used as a sample monograph. (For more information about other opioids molecules, please refer to the FDA website at *www.accessdata.fda.gov/scripts/cder/daf.*)

Oxycodone (Immediate Release)
Tablets: 5 mg, 10 mg, 15 mg, 20 mg, 30 mg
Liquid: 1 mg/mL, 20 mg/mL

ORAL CONDITIONS	• Dental pain management
SAMPLE PRESCRIPTION	• Take 1 to 2 tablets (1x 5 mg to 2x 5 mg) every 4 to 6 hours for 4 days as needed for pain (16-48 tablets)

BLACK BOX WARNING

Addiction, abuse, and misuse: assess each patient's risk factors and monitor regularly.

Life-threatening respiratory depression: monitor for respiratory depression, especially during initiation of treatment or following a dose increase.

Accidental ingestion: accidental ingestion of oxycodone especially by children, can result in a fatal overdose.

Neonatal opioid withdrawal syndrome: prolonged use of oxycodone or hydrocodone during pregnancy can result in neonatal opioid withdrawal syndrome.

Cytochrome P450 3A4 interaction: the concomitant use of oxycodone with all cytochrome P450 3A4 inhibitors may result in an increase in plasma concentrations. In addition, discontinuation of a concomitantly used cytochrome P450 3A4 inducer may result in an increase in oxycodone concentration.

Risks from concomitant use with benzodiazepines or other CNS depressants: concomitant use of opioids with benzodiazepines or other central nervous system depressants, including alcohol, may result in profound sedation, respiratory depression, coma, and death.

CONTRAINDICATIONS	• Known hypersensitivity to oxycodone • Significant respiratory depression • Acute or severe bronchial asthma in an unmonitored setting • Known or suspected gastrointestinal obstruction, including paralytic ileus
CAUTIONS	• Patient with adrenal insufficiency • Patient with severe hypotension • Hepatotoxicity (when combined with acetaminophen) • Intracranial pressure, brain tumors, head injury, or impaired consciousness • Patients with gastrointestinal conditions • Patients with seizure disorders • Withdrawal

Oxycodone (Immediate Release)

Tablets: 5 mg, 10 mg, 15 mg, 20 mg, 30 mg
Liquid: 1 mg/mL, 20 mg/mL

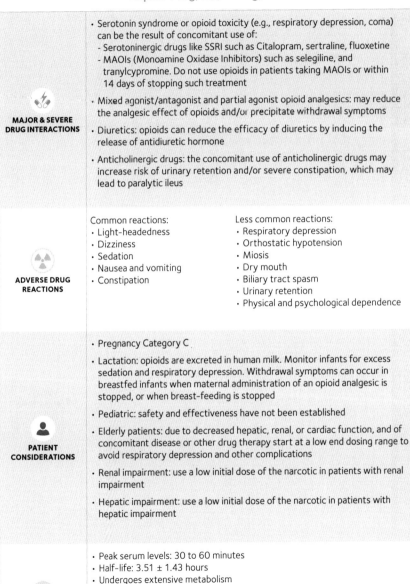

MAJOR & SEVERE DRUG INTERACTIONS

- Serotonin syndrome or opioid toxicity (e.g., respiratory depression, coma) can be the result of concomitant use of:
  - Serotoninergic drugs like SSRI such as Citalopram, sertraline, fluoxetine
  - MAOIs (Monoamine Oxidase Inhibitors) such as selegiline, and tranylcypromine. Do not use opioids in patients taking MAOIs or within 14 days of stopping such treatment
- Mixed agonist/antagonist and partial agonist opioid analgesics: may reduce the analgesic effect of opioids and/or precipitate withdrawal symptoms
- Diuretics: opioids can reduce the efficacy of diuretics by inducing the release of antidiuretic hormone
- Anticholinergic drugs: the concomitant use of anticholinergic drugs may increase risk of urinary retention and/or severe constipation, which may lead to paralytic ileus

ADVERSE DRUG REACTIONS

Common reactions:
- Light-headedness
- Dizziness
- Sedation
- Nausea and vomiting
- Constipation

Less common reactions:
- Respiratory depression
- Orthostatic hypotension
- Miosis
- Dry mouth
- Biliary tract spasm
- Urinary retention
- Physical and psychological dependence

PATIENT CONSIDERATIONS

- Pregnancy Category C
- Lactation: opioids are excreted in human milk. Monitor infants for excess sedation and respiratory depression. Withdrawal symptoms can occur in breastfed infants when maternal administration of an opioid analgesic is stopped, or when breast-feeding is stopped
- Pediatric: safety and effectiveness have not been established
- Elderly patients: due to decreased hepatic, renal, or cardiac function, and of concomitant disease or other drug therapy start at a low end dosing range to avoid respiratory depression and other complications
- Renal impairment: use a low initial dose of the narcotic in patients with renal impairment
- Hepatic impairment: use a low initial dose of the narcotic in patients with hepatic impairment

DRUG CONSIDERATIONS

- Peak serum levels: 30 to 60 minutes
- Half-life: 3.51 ± 1.43 hours
- Undergoes extensive metabolism
- Excretion primarily in urine

Table 3. Sample prescriptions* for the most commonly used opioid analgesics and their combinations**

Opioid	Single-agent	with Acetaminophen (APAP)†	with Aspirin (ASA)	with Ibuprofen	Schedule	Liquid Forms
Codeine		Codeine/APAP (15 mg/300 mg): 1 tablet every 4 to 6 hours as needed (24 tablets) Codeine/APAP (30 mg/300 mg): 1 tablet every 4 to 6 hours as needed (24 tablets) Codeine/APAP (60 mg/300 mg): 1 tablet every 4 to 6 hours as needed (24 tablets)	Codeine/ASA (30 mg/325 mg): 1-2 tablets every 4 hours as needed (48 tablets) Codeine/ASA (60 mg/325 mg): 1 tablet every 4 hours as needed (24 tablets)		Schedule III	Codeine/APAP (12 mg/120 mg) in 5 mL solution Schedule V
Dihydrocodeine			Dihydrocodeine / ASA/ Caffeine (16 mg/ 356.4 mg/ 30 mg) 2 tablets every 4 hours as needed (48 tablets)		Schedule III	
Hydrocodone		Hydrocodone/APAP (5 mg/300 mg) 1-2 tablets every 6 hours as needed (32 tablets)		Hydrocodone/ Ibuprofen (7.5 mg/200 mg) 1 tablet every 4 to 6 hours as needed (32 tablets)	Schedule II	Hydrocodone/APAP (7.5 mg/325 mg) in 15 mL solution Hydrocodone/APAP (10 mg/325 mg) in 15 mL solution

Table 3. Sample prescriptions* for the most commonly used opioid analgesics and their combinations**

Opioid	Single-agent	with Acetaminophen (APAP)†	with Aspirin (ASA)	with Ibuprofen	Schedule	Liquid Forms
Hydromorphone	Hydromorphone 2 mg 1-2 tablets every 4 to 6 hours as needed (48 tablets)				Schedule II	Hydromorphone (5 mg) in 5 mL solution
Oxycodone	Oxycodone IR 5 mg 1-2 tablets every 4 to 6 hours as needed (48 tablets)	Oxycodone/APAP (5 mg/325 mg) 1-2 tablets every 4 to 6 hours as needed (48 tablets)	Oxycodone/ASA (5 mg/325 mg) 1 tablet every 6 hours as needed (16 tablets)	Oxycodone/ibuprofen (5 mg/400 mg) 1 tablet every 6 hours as needed (16 tablets)	Schedule II	Oxycodone/APAP (5 mg/325 mg) in 5 mL solution
Tramadol	Tramadol 50 mg 1-2 tablets every 4 to 6 hours as needed (48 tablets) (max 400 mg/D)	Tramadol/APAP (37.5 mg/325 mg) 1-2 tablets every 4-6 hours as needed (48 tablets)			Schedule IV	

* The sample prescriptions in this handbook represent a general recommendation. Clinicians are responsible to adjust the prescription dose, frequency and length of treatment based on the procedure performed, the medicine prescribed, and the patient conditions such as age, weight, metabolism, liver and renal function.

** Each prescription reflects a 4 days' supply post dental procedure. (Maximum number of tablets displayed in table) The length and frequency of treatment varies on the intensity of the pain, and the medical condition of each patient. Prescriber to use clinical judgment. Extended release formulations not included.

† Remind patient not to take OTC products containing acetaminophen while on opioids combined with APAP (maximum APAP dose 4,000 mg per day). Examples: OTC cough and cold preparations, OTC sleep aids, OTC headache, etc.

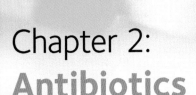

Chapter 2:
Antibiotics

Jay Elkareh, PharmD, PhD

Overview

Orofacial infections are considered mixed infections; they may be caused by either aerobic and anaerobic bacteria or a combination of both. Aerobic bacteria, which require oxygen to survive, include species such as: *Streptococcus viridans* group, *Streptococcus milleri* group, beta-hemolytic streptococcus, *Staphylococcus aureus*, and *Staphylococcus epidermis*. They can be found in plaque, saliva and other locations in the mouth. On the other hand, anaerobic bacteria do not require oxygen to grow and are often isolated in areas like chronic abscess sites. These bacteria include the following species: *Actinomyces, Bacteroides, Eikenella, Fusobacterium, Peptostreptococcus, Prevotella, Porphyromonas,* and *Veillonella*.

1 | Common Indications in Dentistry

Usually, antibiotics are not recommended if the infection is localized, when the patient has a strong immune system, and as a routine prophylaxis measure. (For more information on endocarditis prophylaxis and prosthetic joint infection prophylaxis, refer to section 4: Special Care Patients). When needed, antibiotic treatment must be tailored to each individual case. For instance, an abscessed region will require a different plan of treatment than a systemic infection. While penicillin is the drug of choice for treatment of most empirical infections in and around the oral cavity, other options may need to be considered depending on a patient's response to the regimen. For example, amoxicillin is better absorbed and tolerated by many patients due to a greater bioavailability and less frequent adverse effects like gastrointestinal upset. For patients allergic to penicillin, clindamycin, azithromycin, or metronidazole may serve as an appropriate alternative. On the other hand, in cases where the patient is not allergic to penicillin but is not responding to first line treatment, adding metronidazole to the regimen or substituting amoxicillin with amoxicillin – clavulanic acid may be a good alternative as the spectrum of sensitivity is altered. The clinician is encouraged to culture oral infection followed by antibiotic sensitivity testing, especially for patients who do not respond to the initial course of antibiotic.

2 | Antibiotic Interaction with Oral Contraceptives

In the past, dental practitioners were encouraged to talk to all women of child-bearing age about the possible reduction in efficacy of oral steroid contraceptives during antibiotic therapy. However, new studies have shown no significant drug–drug interaction between hormonal contraceptives and non-rifamycin antibiotics. Simmons et al. in a 2017 systematic review concluded that the evidence from clinical studies outcomes does not support the existence of drug interaction between non-rifamycin antibiotics and hormonal contraceptives (see Suggested Reading List). As a matter of fact, no significant decrease in progestin levels were observed during antibiotic administration. The dentist should advise their patients to use additional protection where the contraceptive pill effectiveness is compromised in instances such as diarrhea or vomiting, caused by either illness or adverse reaction to the antibiotic.

3 | Antibiotic Selection

An antibiotic can come from natural sources, or it can be semi- or totally synthetic. Regardless of the source, antibiotics are classified as either bactericidal or bacteriostatic. Bactericidal drugs directly kill an infecting organism. These include: beta-lactams (penicillins, cephalosporins, carbapenems, monobactams), metronidazole, fluoroquinolones (ciprofloxacin, levofloxacin, moxifloxacin), vancomycin, and aminoglycosides. Bacteriostatic drugs inhibit the proliferation of bacteria by interfering with an essential metabolic process, resulting in the elimination of bacteria by the host's immune defense system. The following drugs are bacteriostatic: tetracyclines (doxycycline, minocycline), macrolides (azithromycin, erythromycin, and clarithromycin), sulfa antibiotics, and clindamycin. In general, there is no advantage in selecting a bactericidal rather than a bacteriostatic antibiotic for the treatment of healthy people. However, if the patient is immunocompromised, either by concurrent treatment (such as cancer chemotherapy or drugs associated with a bone-marrow transplant) or by a preexisting disease (such as HIV infection), a bactericidal antibiotic would be indicated. In general, bactericidal antibiotics should not be used concomitantly with bacteriostatic agents since they may decrease the activity of each.

Over time, the susceptibility of oral bacteria to antibiotics has changed. For example, many gram-positive aerobes and gram-negative anaerobes have shown increased resistance to penicillin. Likewise, aerobic and anaerobic bacteria have developed resistance to some clindamycin regimens. Antibiotic stewardship can limit the development of resistant organisms and enhance patient outcomes. Stewardship emphasizes the responsible use of antibiotics through:

- Identifying the circumstances when antibiotics are indicated
- Choosing the right antibiotic
- Prescribing the right dose and the right duration of therapy

A comprehensive evaluation of every patient is necessary. This involves an assessment of the patient's medical history, then a clinical examination of the infection site, surgical intervention if needed, administration of a suitable antibiotic, and referral to a specialist if necessary.

Antibiotic treatments range from five to seven days on average or three days after the patient's symptoms have subsided. The tables in this chapter will provide information about the most frequently prescribed antibiotics in the dental office.

Antibiotic selection depends on:

- Oral condition-specific determinations such as topical treatment, systemic treatment, or general prophylaxis
- Drug-specific determinations such as the current list of medications the patient is taking, potential drug-drug interactions, and possible side effects/contraindications to the drug to be prescribed
- Patient-specific determinations such as age of the patient, pregnancy/breastfeeding status, or any condition that leaves patient medically compromised
- Antibiotic-specific determinations affecting drug compliance such as length of treatment, frequency of dosage, dosage form, cost of the antibiotic, availability of a generic/brand name option on the formulary

Suggested Reading List

- Ciancio S, ed. ADA/PDR Guide to dental therapeutics. Fifth ed. Chicago: American Dental Association, 2009.
- Flynn TR. What are the antibiotics of choice for odontogenic infections, and how long should the treatment course last? Oral Maxillofac Surg Clin North Am 2011;23(4):519-36.
- Holmes CJ, Pellecchia R. Antimicrobial therapy in management of odontogenic infections in general dentistry. Dent Clin North Am 2016;60(2):497-507.
- Roberts RM, Bartoces M, Thompson SE, Hicks LA. Antibiotic prescribing by general dentists in the United States, 2013. J Am Dent Assoc 2017;148(3):172-78.e1.
- Segura-Egea JJ, Gould K, Sen BH, et al. Antibiotics in endodontics: a review. Int Endod J 2016: 20(6):1133-41.
- Simmons KB, Haddad LB, Nanda K, Curtis KM, et al Drug interactions between non-rifamycin antibiotics and hormonal contraception: A systematic review. Am J Obstet Gynecol. 2017 Jul 7. pii: S0002-9378(17)308-45.

Drug Monograph

The following tables list some of the antibiotics commonly used in dentistry.

In the monographs below, prophylaxis includes prosthetic joint infection prophylaxis or endocarditis prophylaxis. The most current guidelines are available at *ebd.ada.org*.

NOTE: The sample prescriptions in this handbook represent a general recommendation. Clinicians are responsible to adjust the prescription dose, frequency and length of treatment based on the procedure performed, the medicine prescribed, and the patient conditions such as age, weight, metabolism, liver and renal function.

Amoxicillin – A Penicillin

Tablet/Capsule: 250 mg, 500 mg, 875 mg · Chewable tablets: 125 mg, 250 mg
Liquid: 125 mg/5 mL, 200 mg/5 mL, 250 mg/5 mL, 400 mg/5 mL

ORAL CONDITIONS	• Acute oral infection • Sinusitis • Prophylaxis
SAMPLE PRESCRIPTION	• Take 1 tablet (500 mg) 3 times a day for 5 to 7 days (15-21 tablets) • For prophylaxis, take 4 tablets (4x 500 mg) 1 hour before dental procedure (4 tablets)
CONTRAINDICATIONS	• Hypersensitivity to penicillin
⚠ **CAUTIONS**	• Hypersensitivity to cephalosporins, carbapenem, imipenem • Superinfection may occur with prolonged use • Previously confirmed C. difficile-assoc. diarrhea • Patient with infectious mononucleosis

MAJOR & SEVERE DRUG INTERACTIONS	• This drug ↓ the effect of live vaccines such as BCG, cholera, typhoid
	• This drug ↑ the concentration of methotrexate
	• The following medications may ↓ the therapeutic effects of this drug:
	  - Tetracycline such as minocycline, doxycycline, demeclocycline
	  - Gastroesophageal drugs such as esomeprazole, lansoprazole, dexilansoprazole, omeprazole, pantoprazole
	  - GLP-1 receptor agonist antidiabetic medications such as exenatide, and lixisenatide
	• Aminoglycosides such as amikacin, gentamicin, streptomycin, tobramycin ↑ the concentration, efficacy and bactericidal effects of this drug

☢ **ADVERSE DRUG REACTIONS**	Common reactions: • Nausea, vomiting, diarrhea • Urticaria, rash • Black hairy tongue • Oral or vaginal candidiasis Less common reactions: • Anaphylaxis, Stevens-Johnson syndrome, toxic epidermal necrolysis • C. difficile-assoc. diarrhea, hepatitis
PATIENT CONSIDERATIONS	• Pregnancy Category B • Lactation: drug enters breast milk; use with caution • Adjust dose and frequency of drug to twice a day or daily based on severity of renal impairment • No hepatic dose adjustment needed
DRUG CONSIDERATIONS	• Peak serum time: 2 hr, 1 hr (suspension) • Protein bound: 17-20% • Bioavailability: 74-92% • Half-life: 0.7-1.4 hr • Excretion: urine (60% unchanged drug)

Combination Drug (Amoxicillin – Clavulanate)*

Tablet: 250 mg/125 mg, 500 mg/125 mg, 875 mg/125 mg
Chewable tablets: 200 mg/28.5 mg, 400 mg/57 mg
Liquid: (125 mg/31.25 mg)/5 mL, (200 mg/28.5 mg)/5 mL, (250 mg/62.5 mg)/5 mL, (400 mg/57 mg)/5 mL, (600 mg/42.9 mg)/5 mL

SAMPLE PRESCRIPTION	• Take 1 tablet (500 mg/125 mg) 3 times a day for 5 to 7 days (15-21 tablets)

* Amoxicillin – Clavulanate shares several pharmacological similarities with Amoxicillin, however refer to the drug package insert or the U.S. Food & Drug Administration (*www.fda.gov*), for a complete drug profile for this medication.

Azithromycin – A Macrolide

Tablet: 250 mg, 500 mg
Liquid: 100 mg/5 mL, 200 mg/5 mL

ORAL CONDITIONS	• Acute oral infection • Sinusitis • Prophylaxis
Rx SAMPLE PRESCRIPTION	• Take 2 tablets (500 mg) on day 1, then 1 tablet on days 2 to 5 (6 tablets) • For prophylaxis, take 2 tablets (2x 250 mg) 1 hour before dental procedure (2 tablets)
CONTRAINDICATIONS	• Azithromycin hypersensitivity • Hepatic impairment or cholestatic jaundice • Co-administration of antipsychotic drug; pimozide
CAUTIONS	• Patient with uncompensated heart failure, bradarrythmias, history of torsades de pointes, and unknown prolonged QT intervals • Patients with abnormal liver functions, hepatitis • Patients with myasthenia gravis • Previously confirmed C. difficile-assoc. diarrhea

MAJOR & SEVERE DRUG INTERACTIONS	• This drug ↓ the effect of live vaccines such as BCG, cholera, typhoid
	• This drug ↑ the risk of bleeding with concomitant usage of warfarin
	• This drug ↑ the concentration of cholesterol lowering drugs such as statins
	• This drug when taken with the following drugs ↑ the QTc interval:
	  - Antibiotics such as ciprofloxacin, levofloxacin, moxifloxacin
	  - Narcotics such as hydrocodone, methadone, buprenorphine
	  - Antipsychotics such as thioridazine, pimozide
	  - Antiarrhythmic medications such as dronedarone, amiodarone, procainamide
	  - Antifungals such as fluconazole

ADVERSE DRUG REACTIONS	Common reactions: • Diarrhea, nausea, vomiting • Dizziness, headache, anorexia • Rash, pruritus, vaginitis • Impaired hearing with high doses used Less common reactions: • Angioedema, Stevens-Johnson syndrome, anaphylaxis • Hepatotoxicity, pancreatitis, cholestatic jaundice • Infantile hypertrophic pyloric stenosis • Torsades de pointes, QT prolongation • Myasthenia gravis exacerbation
PATIENT CONSIDERATIONS	• Pregnancy Category B • Lactation: drug enters breast milk; not recommended • No renal or hepatic dose adjustment needed • Take on an empty stomach
DRUG CONSIDERATIONS	• Peak serum time: 2-3 hr • Bioavailability: 37% • Protein bound: 7-50% • Half-life: 70 hr • Excretion: feces (50%), urine (5-12%)

Clindamycin – A Lincosamide
Tablet: 150 mg, 300 mg · Liquid: 75 mg/5 mL

ORAL CONDITIONS

- Acute oral infection
- Prophylaxis

SAMPLE PRESCRIPTION

- Take 1 tablet (150 mg) 4 times per day for 7-10 days (28-40 tablets)
- For prophylaxis, take 4 tablets (4x 150 mg) 1 hour before procedure (4 tablets)

BLACK BOX WARNING – C. difficile-assoc. diarrhea (CDAD) has been reported and may range in severity from mild diarrhea to fatal colitis. Caution is recommended when prescribing this drug to patients with a history of CDAD or gastro-intestinal disorders.

CONTRAINDICATIONS

- Hypersensitivity to clindamycin, lincomycin

CAUTIONS

- Patients with hepatic or renal impairment

MAJOR & SEVERE DRUG INTERACTIONS

- This drug ↓ the effect of:
  - Antibiotics such as erythromycin
  - Live vaccines such as BCG, cholera, typhoid
- This drug ↑ the concentration and respiratory depression of Neuromuscular blocking agents such as succinylcholine, onabotulinumtoxinA, vecuronium

ADVERSE DRUG REACTIONS

Common reactions:
- Rash, urticaria, pruritus
- Diarrhea, nausea, vomiting
- Hypotension, jaundice
- Metallic taste

Less common reactions:
- Anaphylaxis, Stevens-Johnson syndrome, toxic epidermal necrolysis
- C. difficile-assoc. diarrhea, fungal overgrowth
- Renal impairment, vaginitis

PATIENT CONSIDERATIONS

- Pregnancy Category B
- Lactation: excreted in breast milk; compatible with breastfeeding
- Monitor patients with renal impairment
- Monitor patients with hepatic impairment
- May take with food

DRUG CONSIDERATIONS

- Peak serum time: 1-3 hr
- Bioavailability: 90%
- Half-life: 2-3 hr
- Excretion: urine (10%), feces (4%)

Doxycycline – A Tetracycline

Tablet: 20 mg, 50 mg, 75 mg, 100 mg, 150 mg • Liquid: 25 mg/5 mL

 ORAL CONDITIONS	• Periodontal disease • Sinusitis
 SAMPLE PRESCRIPTION	• Take 1 tablet (100 mg) twice a day the 1st day, then 1 tablet (100 mg) daily for 4 to 6 additional days (6-8 tablets) • For chronic periodontitis, take 1 tablet (20 mg) 2 times a day for up to 9 months following scaling and root planing
 CONTRAINDICATIONS	• Allergies to tetracycline
 CAUTIONS	• Pediatric patients due to possible permanent tooth discoloration • Superficial discoloration of adult dentin, reversible after drug discontinuation and dental cleaning • Previous confirmed C. difficile-assoc. diarrhea • Patients with history with intracranial hypertension

MAJOR & SEVERE DRUG INTERACTIONS
	• This drug ↓ the effect of:
	  – Live vaccines such as BCG, cholera, typhoid
	  – Penicillin family of drugs due to pharmacological competition
	• The drug ↑ the concentration of certain narcotic drugs such as fentanyl
	• The drug ↑ the side effects of retinoic acid derivatives
	• The following family of medications ↓ the concentration and efficacy of Multivitamins and minerals containing vitamins A,D,E,K, folate, or iron

 ADVERSE DRUG REACTIONS	Common reactions: • Dentin and skin discoloration • Rashes, photosensitivity • Headache • Anorexia, nausea, vomiting, diarrhea Less common reactions: • Urticaria, angioneurotic edema, anaphylactoid purpura • Pericarditis, esophagitis, hepatitis, pancreatitis, vasculitis • Hepatotoxicity, nephrotoxicity • Bulging fontanels in infants and intracranial hypertension in adults • Brown-black microscopic discoloration of the thyroid gland when given for a long period of time • Hemolytic anemia, thrombocytopenia, neutropenia
 PATIENT CONSIDERATIONS	• Pregnancy Category D • Lactation: enters breast milk; not recommended • Not recommended for patients < 8 years of age • No renal or hepatic dose adjustment needed • Don't take with food, dairy products or products containing calcium • Don't get prolonged exposure to sunlight or tanning booths • Minocycline can cause permanent discoloration of permanently erupted teeth
DRUG CONSIDERATIONS	• Oral: reduced 20% by food or milk • Peak serum time: 1.5-4 hr • Bioavailability: reduced at high pH • Protein bound: 90% • Half-life: 15-25 hr • Excretion: feces (primary), urine (secondary)

Erythromycin – A Macrolide
Tablet: 250 mg, 500 mg

ORAL CONDITIONS	• Acute oral infection
 **SAMPLE PRESCRIPTION**	• Take 1 tablet (500 mg) 2 times a day for 5 to 7 days (10-14 tablets)
CONTRAINDICATIONS	• Hypersensitivity to macrolides • Patients with migraines taking ergotamine or dihydroergotamine • Patients with previous hepatitis to macrolides • Patients with hepatic impairment
CAUTIONS	• Patients with uncontrolled arrhythmia

MAJOR & SEVERE DRUG INTERACTIONS	• This drug ↓ the effect of:
	  - Live vaccines such as BCG, cholera, typhoid
	  - Sedative barbiturates such as secobarbital, phenobarbital
	  - Blood thinners such as clopidogrel
	• This drug ↑ the concentration of:
	  - Corticosteroids such as prednisone, dexamethasone, triamcinolone
	  - Antianxiolytics such as alprazolam, diazepam, midazolam
	  - Muscle relaxants such as tizanidine
	  - HIV drugs such as lopinavir, tipranavir
	  - Blood thinners such as heparin, warfarin
	  - Narcotics such as fentanyl
	  - Cholesterol lowering drugs such as Statins
	  - Anti-allergy medicine such as loratadine
	  - Antacids such as cimetidine
	  - Asthma medications such as theopylline
	  - Antiarrhythmic medications such as digoxin, verapamil
	
	• The following family of medication ↑ the levels of this drug:
	  - Antifungals such as ketoconazole, voriconazole
	  - Antibiotics such as metronidazole
	  - Migraine and anti-seizure medication such as topiramate
	  - Asthma medications such as zafirlukast
	• This drug when taken with the following drugs ↑ the QTc interval:
	  - Epinephrine
	  - Antibiotics such as clarithromycin, moxifloxacin
	  - Antiemetic such as ondansetron
	  - Antidepressant such as trazodone

ADVERSE DRUG REACTIONS	Common reactions: • Anorexia, diarrhea, nausea, vomiting • Mild allergic reactions, rash • Elevated liver functions ALT, AST, jaundice Less common reactions: • QT prolongation, ventricular arrhythmias • Pancreatitis, hepatitis, pseudomembranous colitis, interstitial nephritis • Myasthenia gravis exacerbation • Hearing loss (reversible) • Anaphylaxis, Stevens-Johnson syndrome, toxic epidermal necrolysis • infantile hypertrophic pyloric stenosis • C. difficile-assoc. diarrhea, hepatitis
PATIENT CONSIDERATIONS	• Pregnancy Category B • Lactation: drug enters breast milk; compatible with breastfeeding • No renal adjustment needed • Not recommended for hepatic impaired patients • Take on an empty stomach
DRUG CONSIDERATIONS	• Peak serum time: 4 hr • Protein bound: 73-81% • Enzymes inhibited: CYP1A2, CYP3A4 • Half-life: 1.5-2 hr • Excretion: feces (primarily), urine (secondary)

Metronidazole – A Nitroimidazole
Tablet: 250 mg, 500 mg

ORAL CONDITIONS	• Periodontal disease • Acute dental infection (anaerobes)
SAMPLE PRESCRIPTION	• Take 1 tablet (250 mg) 3 times a day for 7 to 10 days (21-30 tablets)

BLACK BOX WARNING – Carcinogenic risk in small animals such as mice and rats; avoid unnecessary use.

CONTRAINDICATIONS	• Metronidazole or nitroimidazole derivatives hypersensitivity • Pregnancy during their first trimester • Alcohol consumption up to 3 days after end of therapy • Patients being treated with disulfiram in the past two weeks
CAUTIONS	• Encephalopathy, seizures, aseptic meningitis, and peripheral neuropathies may occur with higher doses and chronic therapy • Superinfection may occur with prolonged use

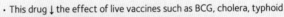 **MAJOR & SEVERE DRUG INTERACTIONS**	• This drug ↓ the effect of live vaccines such as BCG, cholera, typhoid
	• This drug ↑ the concentration of the following drugs:
	  - Blood thinners like warfarin
	  - Antineoplastic drugs such as fluorouracil, carbocisteine, busulfam, and capecitabine
	  - Cholesterol lowering drugs such as lomitapide
	  - Appetite stimulants drugs such as Dronabinol
	• This drug ↑ the effect of alcohol intoxication:
	  - Medication containing alcohol or propylene glycol
	• The following family of medication ↑ the levels of this drug:
	  - Antiseizure drugs such as phentobarbital, phenytoin, primidone
	  - Drugs to treat alcoholism such as disulfiram

ADVERSE DRUG REACTIONS	Common reactions: • Headache, nausea, dizziness • Metallic taste, xerostomia • Vaginitis, genital pruritis • Bacterial infection, candidiasis, sinusitis, pharyngitis Less common reactions: • Seizure, aseptic meningitis, optic neuropathy • Stevens–Johnson syndrome, toxic epidermal necrolysis • Leukopenia, carcinogenicity
PATIENT CONSIDERATIONS	• Pregnancy Category B; however contraindicated in 1st trimester • Lactation: drug enters breast milk; use with caution • No renal or hepatic dose adjustment needed • Don't drink alcohol or take alcohol containing cough syrup while on medication
DRUG CONSIDERATIONS	• Peak serum 1-2 hr • Bioavailability: 80% absorption • Protein bound: < 20% • Enzymes inhibited: CYP2C9 • Half-life: 8 hr • Excretion: feces (14%), urine (77%)

Penicillin VK – A Penicillin
Tablet: 250 mg, 500 mg
Liquid: 125 mg/5 mL, 250 mg/5 mL

ORAL CONDITIONS	• Acute oral infection
SAMPLE PRESCRIPTION	• Take 1 tablet (500 mg) 4 times per day for 5-7 days (20-28 tablets)
CONTRAINDICATIONS	• Penicillin allergies including anaphylaxis • Asthmatic patients prone to allergy
CAUTIONS	• Cephalosporins, carbapenem, imipenem hypersensitivity • Patients with history of antibiotic associated colitis

MAJOR & SEVERE DRUG INTERACTIONS	• The following medications ↓ the concentration and efficacy of this drug:
	  - Tetracycline such as minocycline, doxycycline, demeclocycline
	  - Gastroesophageal drugs such as esomeprazole, lansoprazole, dexilansoprazole, omeprazole, pantoprazole
	  - GLP-1 receptor agonist antidiabetic medications such as exenatide, and lixisenatide
	• Aminoglycosides such as amikacin, gentamicin, streptomycin, tobramycin ↑ the concentration, efficacy and bactericidal effects of this drug
	• This drug ↓ the effect of live vaccines such as BCG, cholera, typhoid
	• This drug ↑ the concentration of methotrexate

ADVERSE DRUG REACTIONS	Common reactions: • Nausea, vomiting, diarrhea • Candidiasis, and other fungal infections Less common reactions: • C. difficile-assoc. diarrhea • Anemia, positive Coombs reaction, bleeding • Interstitial nephritis • Hypersensitivity
PATIENT CONSIDERATIONS	• Pregnancy Category B • Lactation: excreted in breast milk; compatible with breastfeeding • No renal or hepatic dose adjustment needed, however, monitor patients with renal impairment • Take on an empty stomach
DRUG CONSIDERATIONS	• Bioavailability: 60-73% • Peak serum time: 0.5-1 hr • Protein bound: 80% • Half-life: 0.5-0.6 hr • Excretion: urine

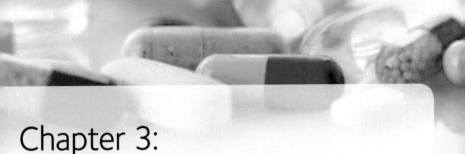

Chapter 3:
Antifungals

S. Craig Rhodes, DMD, MSD

Overview

Fungal infections encountered in dental practice can vary from being superficial to deep. Whether presenting as a local manifestation, or as a symptom of a systemic infection, it is important for all dental clinicians to familiarize themselves with the common presentations and treatment alternatives for oral fungal infections.

NOTE: The sample prescriptions in this handbook represent a general recommendation. Clinicians are responsible to adjust the prescription dose, frequency and length of treatment based on the procedure performed, the medicine prescribed, and the patient conditions such as age, weight, metabolism, liver and renal function.

1 | Oral Candidiasis

Candida is a dimorphic organism normally found in the gastrointestinal and vaginal tracts of humans. The fungus is dimorphic, existing in a yeast as well as a hyphal phase. The presence of Candida in and on the human body is typically well tolerated, and the organism is not normally viewed as being pathogenic.

The situation can change when the normal environment is interrupted from conditions and practices such as: immune system compromise, a breach in the mucosa or skin, decreases in salivary flow (xerostomia), the introduction of dental prostheses such as acrylic dentures, nutritional deficiencies, the use of broad-spectrum antibiotics and the intake of other medications, such as chronically-administered steroids.

It is important to replace contaminated oral hygiene devices (toothbrushes, denture brushes) to prevent relapse of the infection after successful treatment. It is highly recommended for patients on continuous positive airway pressure (CPAP) therapy to follow strict hygiene guidelines to prevent fungal contamination, and further systemic infection. Oral fungal infections can be localized or associated with systemic infection.

Table 1. Superficial Oral Fungal Infections

Pseudomembranous Candidiasis (Thrush)

Clinical Picture	• Most commonly seen form of oral fungal infection caused by *Candida* (35%) • Clinical predictor of HIV disease progression • Presents with a white, "cottage cheese" appearance that often, when scraped off, typically leaves a raw, erythematous surface that can bleed easily • Can present with oral burning sensation and/or sense of taste abnormalities

Affected Populations	• The very young and the very old (populations having immune system deficiencies)
	• People who are immunocompromised, often as resulting from disease or certain medications such as:
	  – Broad-spectrum antibiotics
	  – Prednisone
	  – Inhaled corticosteroids
	  – Drugs that cause dry mouth

Drugs of Choice*	• Clotrimazole troche
	  – Disp: 70 troches
	  – Sig: Dissolve 1 troche in the mouth 5 times/day until gone
	  – Advise the patient to allow the troche 15–30 minutes to dissolve in the mouth
	  – Troches contain sucrose and can increase caries risk with prolonged use (> 3 months) and dry mouth conditions
	• Nystatin tablets
	  – Disp: 30 tablets
	  – Sig: Dissolve 1 tablet in the mouth, 4 times/day
	• Nystatin suspension
	  – Disp: 300 mL
	  – Sig: Swish with 1 tsp 4 times/day and expectorate
	  – Suspension vehicle contains 50% sucrose and can increase caries risk with prolonged use (>3 months) and/or dry mouth conditions
	• Fluconazole – to be used only if infection does not respond to the Clotrimazole or Nystatin
	  – Disp: 16 tablets
	  – Sig: Take 2 tablets on day one and 1 tablet/day thereafter until resolved
	  – Take for 14 days

* Also, see the drug monograph for Clotrimazole, Nystatin, and Fluconazole at the end of the chapter.

Table 1. Superficial Oral Fungal Infections

Erythematous Candidiasis (Atrophic)

Clinical Picture	• Absence of a pseudomembranous coating
	• Areas most affected:
	  - Palate – erythematous patches
	  - Dorsum of the tongue (median rhomboid glossitis), results in depappillation, and affects 3 times more men than women
	  - Corners of the mouth
	• Most often associated with the use of broad-spectrum antibiotics or corticosteroids
	• Raw-looking appearance
	• Painful

Chronic Hyperplastic Candidiasis

Clinical Picture	• Also known as candida leukoplakia since there is a white plaque present
	• Areas most affected:
	  - Commissural region of the buccal mucosa
	  - Palate
	  - Tongue
	• Cannot be readily wiped away
	• Is often associated with a diagnosis of epithelial dysplasia
	• Close follow-up is advised, especially if the lesions are recalcitrant to therapy, and a tissue biopsy may be indicated to determine if dysplasia is present

Table 1. Superficial Oral Fungal Infections	
Angular Cheilitis (Perleche)	

Clinical Picture	• A form of chronic atrophic candidiasis
	• A mixed bacterial-fungal infection
	• Erythematous fissures develop at the commissures, often covered with a pseudomembranous coating and/or a crusting/scaling appearance
	• May also affect the anterior portion of the nares
	• Requires a moist environment
	• Symptoms can range from asymptomatic to severe discomfort, itching, burning, irritation
	• Contributing factors include:
	  - Reduced vertical dimension of occlusion – ill-fitting dentures
	  - Facial wrinkling along nasolabial folds or corners of the mouth
	  - Thumb sucking
	  - Tobacco smoking
	  - Down syndrome
	  - Hypersalivation
	  - HIV
	  - Solid organ cancer (pancreas, kidney, liver)
	  - Medical conditions: anemia, diabetes
	  - Nutritional deficiencies: iron, thiamine, riboflavin, folic acid

Affected Populations	• Patients who wear dentures having a reduced vertical dimension of occlusion • Patients with increased wrinkling or folding of skin at the corners of the mouth • Patients with diabetes, immunological disorders, solid organ cancer, hematologic malignancies, nutritional deficiencies

Drugs of Choice*	• Combination of a topical antifungal and antibacterial (Nystatin and Mupirocin)
	  - Nystatin ointment: 15g or 30g tube – apply to affected areas 2-3 times/day
	  - Mupirocin ointment: 22g tube – apply to affected area 3 times/day
	• Combination of a topical antifungal and glucocorticoid (Nystatin and Triamcinolone)
	  - Nystatin and Triamcinolone cream: 15g tube – apply to affected area 2-4 times/day

* Also, see the drug monograph for Nystatin at the end of the chapter.

Table 1. Superficial Oral Fungal Infections

Denture-Associated Stomatitis

Clinical Picture	• A form of chronic atrophic candidiasis
	• Also known as denture sore mouth
	• Porosity of the denture and moist environment allows for fungal and bacterial contamination
	• Three progressive stages:
	  1. Palatal petechiae
	  2. Diffuse erythema involving most of the mucosa covered by the denture
	  3. Development of tissue granulation (papillary hyperplasia)
	• Any treatment must be accompanied by thorough disinfection of the denture or reoccurrence of the infection is likely to happen
	  – 10 minute soak in 0.5% household bleach (1 part bleach to 10 parts water) is sufficient. Do not soak the prosthesis in bleach overnight.

Affected Populations	• Patients who wear dentures

Drugs of Choice (if disinfection of the denture prosthesis and/or correction of the denture deficiencies are insufficient)*	• Clotrimazole troche
	  – Disp: 70 troches
	  – Sig: Dissolve 1 troche in the mouth 5 times/day until troches are gone
	  – Advise the patient to allow the troche 15–30 minutes to dissolve in the mouth
	  – Troches contain sucrose and can increase caries risk with prolonged use (>3 months) and/or dry mouth conditions
	• Chlorhexidine gluconate oral rinse 0.12%
	  – Disp: 3x 16 oz
	  – Sig: swish with 15 mL (1 capful) undiluted oral rinse for 30 seconds, then expectorate. Caution patient against swallowing the medicine and advise no eating for 2–3 hours after treatment.

Central Papillary Atrophy (Median Rhomboid Glossitis)

Clinical Picture	• Relatively uncommon (prevalence is less than 1%) • Typically has been associated with a chronic Candida infection, although the importance of the Candida as an etiologic agent is unknown at the present time • Lesion may not resolve completely with antifungal therapy • 3:1 male-female incidence ratio

* Also, see the drug monograph for Clotrimazole at the end of the chapter.

2 | Deep-seated Fungal Oral Infections (possibly associated with systemic disease)

Oral fungal infections can be localized or associated with systemic infection such as histoplasmosis typically presented as a single ulcerated lesion. Mucormycosis usually presented as a palatal ulceration can lead to brain necrosis if not treated. While blastomycosis produces ulceration of the oral mucosa, cryptococcosis rarely produces ulcerations that are superficial in nature. Both seen primarily in immunocompromised patients, aspergillosis causes black or yellow palatal lesions by extension from the maxillary sinus, and geotrichosis produces mucosal lesions that can be covered by a pseudomembrane, similar to pseudomembranous candidiasis, for which it is often mistaken. When systemic fungal infection is suspected, consider referring patient to appropriate specialist.

📖 | Suggested Reading List

- Ciancio SG, ed. ADA/PDR Guide to Dental Therapeutics. 5th edition. Chicago: American Dental Association/Physicians' Desk Reference, Inc.; 2009.
- Jacobsen PL. The Little Dental Drug Booklet 2016-2017. Lexicomp. Wolters Kluwer; 2016.
- Jeske A. Mosby's Dental Drug Reference. 12th edition. St. Louis: Mosby; 2017.
- Muzyka BC, Epifanio RN. Update on oral fungal infections. Dent Clin North Am 2013;57(4):561-81.
- Telles Dr, Karki N, Marshall MW. Oral fungal infections diagnosis and management. Dent Clin North Am 2017;61(2):319-49.

Drug Monograph

The following tables list some of the most commonly used antifungals in dentistry today.

NOTE: The sample prescriptions in this handbook represent a general recommendation. Clinicians are responsible to adjust the prescription dose, frequency and length of treatment based on the procedure performed, the medicine prescribed, and the patient conditions such as age, weight, metabolism, liver and renal function.

Clotrimazole
Troche: 10 mg

ORAL CONDITIONS	• Candidiasis Oropharyngeal
SAMPLE PRESCRIPTION	• Dissolve 1 troche (10 mg) in the mouth 5 times per day for 15-30 minutes until troches are gone (70 troches)
CONTRAINDICATIONS	• Hypersensitivity • Patients on cisapride, or lomitapide
CAUTIONS	• Patients with liver impairment, monitor liver function tests

MAJOR & SEVERE DRUG INTERACTIONS	• This drug ↑ the concentration and toxic side effects of the following:
	  - Cisapride, lomitapide (contraindication)
	  - Opioids such as codeine, methadone, hydrocodone, oxycodone
	  - Blood thinners such as warfarin
	  - Antidiabetics such as glyburide, glipizide
	  - Hyperlipidemia drugs such as simvastatin, atorvastatin
	  - Antibiotics such as erythromycin
	• This drug ↓ the concentration and efficacy of the following:
	  - Antibiotics such as azithromycin
	  - Antiarrhythmic such as digoxin
	  - Corticosteroids such as prednisone, dexamethasone

ADVERSE DRUG REACTIONS	Common reactions: • Abnormal liver function tests • Nausea, vomiting
PATIENT CONSIDERATIONS	• Pregnancy Category C • Lactation: unknown if excreted in breast milk; caution recommended with breastfeeding
DRUG CONSIDERATIONS	• Bioavailability: poor absorption • Metabolism: liver • Half-life: unknown • Excretion: feces (100%)

Fluconazole
Tablet: 50 mg, 100 mg, 150 mg, 200 mg
Liquid: 10 mg/mL, 40 mg/mL

ORAL CONDITIONS	• Candidiasis Oropharyngeal • Candidiasis Systemic
Rx **SAMPLE PRESCRIPTION**	• Take 2 Tablets (2x 100 mg) on day 1, then 1 (100 mg) tablet daily for 14 days (16 tablets) • For candidemia, take 8 (8x 100 mg) Tablets on day 1, then 4 (4x 100 mg) tablets daily for 14 days (64 tablets) (off-label use)
CONTRAINDICATIONS	• Azole hypersensitivity • Pregnancy • Patients with congenital long QT • Patients taking drugs that prolong QT such as erythromycin, quinidine, cisapride
⚠ **CAUTIONS**	• Patients taking warfarin • Patients with hepatic impairment • Patients taking statins
MAJOR & SEVERE DRUG INTERACTIONS	• This drug ↑ the concentration and toxic side effects of the following: - Blood thinners like warfarin, clopidogrel (life threatening drug interaction) - Hyperlipidemia drugs such as simvastatin, lovastatin - Antiarrythmic drugs such as digoxin, quinidine, procainamide, amiodarone - Antibiotics macrolides such as erythromycin, clarithromycin - Antibiotics fluoroquinolones such as moxifloxacin - Narcotics such as tramadol, fentanyl - Benzodiazepines such as alprazolam, diazepam, triazolam - Antimigraine drugs especially the ergotamine family - Epinephrine
☢ **ADVERSE DRUG REACTIONS**	Common reactions: • Nausea, vomiting, diarrhea • Dyspepsia, taste change • Elevated liver function (AST, ALT) Less common reactions: • Anaphylaxis, Stevens–Johnson syndrome, angioedema • Torsade de pointe, QT prolongation • Hepatotoxicity, leukopenia, thrombocytopenia
👤 **PATIENT CONSIDERATIONS**	• Pregnancy Category D • Lactation: excreted in breast milk; caution recommended with breastfeeding • Monitor liver function, renal functions, and potassium levels • Avoid alcohol consumption while on medication
DRUG CONSIDERATIONS	• Bioavailability: > 90% • Peak serum time: 1-2 hr • Protein bound: 11-12% • Metabolism: liver • Half-life: 30 hr • Excretion: urine (80%), metabolites (11%)
ALTERNATIVE DRUG	For Fluconazole-refractory candidiasis use: Voriconazole (200 mg tablets or 200 mg/5 mL liquid): Take 1 Tablet (200 mg) 2 times a day 1 hr before or after meals for 21 days or until infection resolved (42 tablets)

Nystatin
Tablet: 500,000 units
Liquid: 100,000 units/mL
Ointment/cream: 100,000 units/g

ORAL CONDITIONS	• Candidiasis Oropharyngeal
SAMPLE PRESCRIPTION	• Dissolve 1 tablet (500,000 units) in the mouth 4 times per day until troches are gone (30 tablets) • For Angular Cheilitis (Perleche): Apply to affected skin areas 2 to 3 times per day (30 g ointment/cream)
CONTRAINDICATIONS	• Hypersensitivity
CAUTIONS	• Don't use for systemic mycoses
MAJOR & SEVERE DRUG INTERACTIONS	• No significant interactions reported
ADVERSE DRUG REACTIONS	Common reactions: • Nausea, vomiting, diarrhea • Dermatitis Less common reactions: • Stevens-Johnson syndrome
PATIENT CONSIDERATIONS	• Pregnancy Category C • Lactation: unknown if excreted in breast milk; caution recommended with breastfeeding • Symptom relief in 24-72 hours
DRUG CONSIDERATIONS	• Bioavailability: poor absorption • Half-life: unknown • Excretion: feces (100%)

Chapter 4:
Antivirals and Vaccines

Paul Eleazer, DDS, MS

Overview

1 | Antiviral Treatments

Herpes Simplex Virus (Cold Sores)

Cold sores, also known as fever blisters, are the most commonly seen oral viral infection. One of nine known human pathogens in the herpes virus family, HSV-1 causes cold sores that are characterized by an initial infection, with persistence in nerve cell bodies that reside in ganglia. These lesions are contagious, which makes them dangerous to patient and provider.

Treatment

The vesicles rupture about day two, releasing countless viruses. Prompt treatment, ideally at the prodromal stage, with topical or systemic antiviral drugs will mitigate the severity and duration of the outbreak. Treatment might differ based on the severity of the infection and the immunocompetency of the patient. For patients who are immunocompromised, a systemic drug such as acyclovir or valacyclovir is preferred.

In cases of mild infection, a topical prescription form of antiviral medication plus a numbing agent is recommended. Other treatments can be found over-the-counter (OTC) at pharmacies (Refer to table 1 on page 42). Docosanol cream, which is available OTC, provides a barrier that can be helpful. It is notable, however, that this barrier does not prevent viral shedding, thus handwashing and avoiding physical contact with the ulceration remain important. Finally, Benzalkonium chloride combined with benzocaine which is a non-prescription product, is also available from dental supply sources.

Infections around the eyes should be treated by an ophthalmologist. Dental healthcare workers should consider rescheduling a patient with vesicles or draining exudate.

Many additional therapies have been suggested:

- Disinfectants such as Betadine, possibly mixed with alcohol as a drying agent, have proven helpful for some patients. Betadine is an effective disinfectant for the exudate.
- Antimicrobial mouthwashes such as hydrogen peroxide, or chlorhexidine can be used to prevent plaque accumulation especially when brushing is painful.
- Non-pharmacological treatments such as bed rest, increased fluid intake, and avoidance of sun exposure may be helpful.

(**NOTE**: There is a genital strain of the virus, Herpes simplex type 2 (HSV-2), which also can occur orally. It is in another group of the nine member herpes family. Treatment is similar to that of HSV-1.)

Aphthous Ulcers (Canker Sores)

Aphthous ulcers or canker sores are another common oral condition, but are probably not viral in origin. Antiviral therapies are not effective in treating aphthous ulcers. Differentiation from cold sores is important to properly treat these ulcers. Often a traumatic event precedes the prodromal phase, similar to the herpetic eruption. In addition, aphthous ulcers have been associated with the frequent use of NSAIDs.

Aphthous ulcers occur as single or multiple intraoral lesions, generally on non-keratinized mucous membranes and not on attached mucosa, the hard palate or the tongue dorsum. They are not infectious, pointing away from a microbial origin. Also, pointing away from an infectious cause is the fact that they lack a vesicular state. Some have noted that smokers are less likely to experience these lesions, ostensibly due to thicker epithelium.

Treatment

Aphthous ulcers resolve spontaneously but may benefit from topical application of anesthetics or barriers (See Chapter 8: Oral Lesions and Corticosteroids). Many therapies have been suggested for relief of symptoms. There is no vaccine nor curative drug. Specifically, antiviral drugs are not effective. Likewise, antimicrobial agents do not affect these ulcerations, except in preventing secondary infection in patients who are immunocompromised. It has been reported that regular use of the amino acid lysine as a supplement has preventative action. In addition, toothpaste that does not contain sodium lauryl sulfate (SLS) could be recommended to patients with recurrent aphthous ulcers.

Herpes Zoster Virus

The herpes zoster virus causes two relatively common oral conditions, chickenpox and shingles. Like many viral conditions, there is an initial infection (chickenpox), followed by quiescent viral residence within nerve ganglia. Now, many children avoid this problematic disease through vaccination in early childhood. Protection is often not effective for the lifetime of the individual, leading to recurrence in adulthood, known as shingles.

Some evidence exists that people with herpes zoster are more prone to stroke from cerebral infarct.

Treatment

Pain caused by shingles can be extreme, requiring powerful analgesics. Chen et al. performed a meta-analysis that found no effect of acyclovir during treatment at reducing incidence of this pain. Pain apparently is due to nerve damage from the virus. This pain may last for several months. The Centers for Disease Control and Prevention recommends the shingle vaccine (Zostavax) for patients over the age of 60 years of age whether they have had shingles in the past or not. The vaccine has been approved for people over the age of 50 years.

Human Papilloma Virus (HPV)

A member of the herpes family of DNA viruses, the human papilloma virus (HPV) was first associated with cervical cancer; it is now known to cause oropharyngeal cancer. These cancers were once rare but are now relatively more common, especially in young adults due to the increase incidence of oral pharyngeal cancer. (For more information on oral cancer detection and evaluation, see the *ADA Evidence-Based Clinical Practice Guideline for the Evaluation of potential malignant disorders in the oral cavity.* Accessed August 3, 2018.)

Treatment

There is an effective vaccine. This vaccine targets surface proteins and carries no genetic material, thus cannot cause diseases. The vaccine is currently recommend for preteens and young teens prior to sexual activity.

Dentists have an important role in urging parents to have their children vaccinated in their pre-teen and early teen years. One speaker at an ADA seminar suggests that it may be useful to add a question about HPV knowledge on your health questionnaire for all patients.

2 | Vaccination Recommendations

Herpes Zoster Virus

There is a two-dose vaccination available to prevent or minimize the effects of chickenpox (Varivax) in children, although it may not offer lifelong protection against shingles, which could develop later in life. The Centers for Disease Control and Prevention recommends the shingle vaccine (Zostavax) for patients over the age of 60 years of age whether they have had shingles in the past or not. The vaccine has been approved for people over the age of 50 years.

Human Papilloma Virus (HPV)

The vaccine against HPV is currently recommend for preteens and young teens prior to sexual activity. Vaccination of healthcare workers is not currently recommended by the CDC because of the high likelihood that they have already been exposed.

Hepatitis B Virus

Vaccination is very effective against this dangerous disease. Many patients become life-long carriers of the virus. Presently, all healthcare workers are required to be protected from this virus with a three injection series.

Suggested Reading List

- Chen N, Li Q, Yang J, et al. (2014). He L, ed. Antiviral treatment for preventing postherpetic neuralgia. Cochrane Database Systematic Reviews. 2 (2): CD006866. PMID 24500927.

- Hussein AA, Helder MN, de Visscher JG, et al, Global incidence of oral and oropharynx cancer in patients younger than 45 years versus older patients: A systematic review, Eur J Cancer. 2017 Sep; 82:115-27.

- McCarthy JP, Browning WD. Teerlink C, Veit G. Treatment of herpes labialis: Comparison of two OTC drugs and untreated controls. J Esthetic and Restor Dent 2012;24(2):103-9.

- Oliver SE, Unger ER, Lewis R, et al. Prevalence of human papillomavirus among females after vaccine introduction: National Health and Nutrition Examination Survey, United States, 2003-2014. J Infect Dis 2017;216(5):594-603.

Drug Monograph

The following tables list some antivirals commonly used in dentistry today.

NOTE: The sample prescriptions in this handbook represent a general recommendation. Clinicians are responsible to adjust the prescription dose, frequency and length of treatment based on the procedure performed, the medicine prescribed, and the patient conditions such as age, weight, metabolism, liver and renal function.

Acyclovir
Tablets: 200 mg, 400 mg, 800 mg · Liquid: 200 mg/5mL
Topical: see Table 1 on page 42

ValAcyclovir
Tablets: 500 mg, 1000 mg

 ORAL CONDITIONS	· Herpes Simplex Labliasis (cold sores)

SAMPLE PRESCRIPTION
	Acyclovir:
	· Take 1 Tablet (400 mg)
	  3 times per day for 5-10 days
	  (15-30 tablets)
	
	ValAcyclovir:
	· Take 2 Tablets (2x 1000 mg)
	  2 times per day for 1 day
	  (4 tablets)

 CONTRAINDICATIONS	· Acyclovir or valacyclovir hypersensitivity
 CAUTIONS	· Patients with renal failure or renal impairment · Patients with reported thrombocytopenic purpura/hemolytic uremic syndrome

MAJOR & SEVERE DRUG INTERACTIONS
	· This drug ↓ the effect of live vaccines such as Varicella virus vaccine, and Zoster vaccine
	· This drug ↑ the concentration and toxic side effects of the following:
	  - Muscle relaxants such as tizanidine
	  - Immunosuppressive drugs such as mycophenolate
	  - Antipsychotics such as clozapine

 ADVERSE DRUG REACTIONS	Common reactions: · Nausea, vomiting, diarrhea · Photosensitivity, rash · Elevated renal function (creatinine and BUN) Less common reactions: · Anaphylaxis, Stevens-Johnson syndrome, angioedema, erythema multiforme · Hallucination, seizure, encephalopathy · Renal failure, hepatitis, thrombocytopenia · Coma
 PATIENT CONSIDERATIONS	· Pregnancy Category B · Lactation: excreted in breast milk; cautious recommended with breastfeeding · Renal dose adjustment required, avoid concomitant use of other nephrotoxic drugs · No hepatic dose adjustment needed · Resistance for acyclovir has been reported after repeated usage
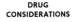 **DRUG CONSIDERATIONS**	**Acyclovir:** · Bioavailability: 60-73% · Absorption: 15-30% · Peak serum time: 1.5-2 hr · Protein bound: 9-33% · Half-life: 3 hr · Excretion: urine (62-90%) **ValAcyclovir:** · Bioavailability: 55% (once converted to Acyclovir) · Peak serum time: Acyclovir is the active drug · Protein bound: 13.5-17.9% · Half-life: 30 min + 3 hr for acyclovir · Excretion: urine (89%), feces (minimal)

Table 1. Topical Antiviral for Cold Sores			
Drug	Indication	Combo	Suggested Directions*
OTC **Docosanol 10% cream (Abreva®)**	Viral Ulceration		Apply 5 times a day up for up to 10 days or until healed
OTC **Benzalkonium chloride 0.13%**	Viral Ulceration/ Pain relief	Benzalkonium chloride 0.13% with Benzocaine 5% or 7.5% (Orajel Single Dose® or Viroxyn®)	Apply once and rub until site becomes numb. Can repeat after 12h if needed
℞ **Penciclovir 1% cream**	Viral Ulceration		Apply every 2 hours while awake for a period of 4 days
℞ **Acyclovir 5% cream**	Viral Ulceration/ Anti-inflammatory	Acyclovir 5% with Hydrocortisone 1% (Xerese®)	Apply 5 times per day for 5 days
℞ **Acyclovir buccal tablets (Sitavig® 50 mg)**	Viral Ulceration		Apply 1 adhesive tablet as a single dose to the upper gum in the canine fossa region: If the tablet falls out or is swallowed within 6 hours apply the 2nd tablet (1 blister package)

* The suggested directions in this handbook represent a general recommendation. Clinicians are responsible to adjust the dose, frequency and length of treatment based on the procedure performed, the medicine prescribed, and the patient conditions such as age, weight, metabolism, liver and renal function.

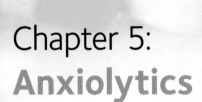

Chapter 5:
Anxiolytics

Elias Mikael Chatah, DMD, BPharm, MS

Overview

1 | Sedative Medications in Dentistry

Nitrous Oxide

Minimal sedation can be achieved with a low-dose oral sedative or nitrous oxide-oxygen inhalation sedation. Nitrous oxide is considered to be a weak anesthetic agent; it is removed from the blood stream via the lungs unchanged, which means that in experienced hands, nitrous oxide is safely administered and the risk of rendering the patient unconscious is small. Nitrous oxide produces relatively weak sedation; as such, it is not recommended for severely anxious or phobic patients.

Doses of nitrous oxide are titrated at 5% increments over 3 to 5 minute intervals; levels up to a maximum of 70% should be sufficient to achieve mild or moderate sedation. Toward the end of the procedure the clinician must titrate nitrous oxide levels down and oxygen levels up until oxygen is administered at 100% for at least five minutes as this decreases the risk for diffusion hypoxia and sudden unconsciousness; at this stage complete recovery ensues and the patient can be discharged in the care of a companion. Patients should be instructed to refrain from having food six hours prior to their appointment as eating increases the risk of emesis during nitrous oxide sedation. As with all sedation techniques, patient consent is required for nitrous sedation.

Nitrous oxide is contraindicated in pregnancy, respiratory infections, chronic obstructive pulmonary disease (COPD), sinus infections, tuberculosis, blocked nasal passages and eustachian tubes, multiple sclerosis and congestive heart failure.

Oral Sedation

Minimal and moderate sedation can be achieved with oral sedation, which involves the oral administration of a sedative agent, the absorption of which occurs in the gastro-intestinal tract. The sedative agent is administered as a premedication, usually one hour prior to the appointment and the night before the appointment. In most cases, sedation that ensues is mild to moderate. Relative to other sedation methods including inhalation and intravenous sedation, oral sedation has a slower onset of action.

Benzodiazepines (BZD)

In the past, clinicians have prescribed antihistamines for anxiety control. However, the current preferred method for oral sedation in dental practice seems to be BZDs, which are psychoactive drugs with anxiolytic, sedative and hypnotic effects. BZDs used in dental practice include alprazolam, clonazepam, diazepam, lorazepam, midazolam, oxazepam and triazolam (Table 1).

Combining nitrous oxide inhalation sedation with higher doses of sedative medication such as BZDs produces moderate and possibly deep sedation; this combination carries a higher risk of respiratory depression. If the clinician chooses this combination, a higher level of patient monitoring is recommended.

For titration guidelines of sedative medication, refer to the "2016 ADA Guidelines for the Use of Sedation and General Anesthesia by Dentists." (see Suggested Reading List on page 48).

2 | Medical Considerations Before Prescribing Benzodiazepines

Prescribing BZDs for anxiety control commands the medical considerations in various patient groups. Refer to Table 2 on page 46.

3 | Pre-Discharge Assessment of Sedation

Following the procedure, the clinician must determine discharge readiness based on the discharge criteria as outlined in the "2016 ADA Guidelines for the Use of Sedation and General Anesthesia by Dentists" (see Suggested Reading List). The half-life of the sedative used must be considered when assessing patients for discharge readiness.

In order to be deemed ready for discharge, patients need to meet the following criteria:
- vital signs within normal limits
- absence of vertigo, nausea and vomiting
- alertness: must be able to state own name, date of birth, address
- orientation to the time, date and place and pre-sedation condition
- ambulation with minimal or no assistance
- presence of a responsible escort who will transport the patient home
- ability to stand unassisted with closed eyes

The time of discharge and the status of the patient at discharge must be documented.

Post-operative instructions must include no alcohol, driving or operating machinery for at least 24 hours following sedation or longer if persistent sedation or drowsiness are experienced.

Table 1. Comparison of Benzodiazepines (BZDs) Used for Dental Anxiety*

Benzodiazepine	Adult Oral Dose (mg)	Onset of Action	Peak Onset (hrs)	Half-life of Parent Drug (hrs)	Active Metabolite	Half-life of Active Metabolite (hrs)
Long Acting						
Diazepam	5	Rapid	1–1.5 (oral)	20–70	Yes	3–100
Intermediate Acting						
Alprazolam	0.5	Intermediate	0.7–1.6	12–18	No	NA
Clonazepam	0.25	Intermediate	1–4	20–40	No	NA
Lorazepam	1	Intermediate	1–1.5 (oral)	10–20	No	NA
Oxazepam	15	Slow	2–3	3–18	No	NA
Short Acting						
Triazolam	0.125–0.25	Intermediate	0.75–2	1–1.5	No	NA

* Do NOT prescribe BZDs in patients taking the following: alcohol, anti-depressants, and opioids. Also, see the drug monograph at the end of the chapter for more information.

Table 2. BZD Risk According to Age, Medical Conditions		
Medical Condition	Benzodiazepine Risk*	Recommendations
Genetic predisposition to addiction	• Slowed metabolizers • Respiratory depression	• Obtain a medical clearance from the patient's physician • Reduce the BZD recommended dose
Alcohol abuse (current or past)	• Serious drug interactions • Respiratory depression • Relapse	Do NOT prescribe BZD
Illicit drug use (current or past)	• Serious drug interactions • Respiratory depression • Relapse	Do NOT prescribe BZD
Drug addiction therapy (e.g., Methadone, Buprenorphine)	• Serious drug interactions • Respiratory depression • Relapse	Do NOT prescribe BZD
Liver pathology	• Excessive sedation • Respiratory depression	• Obtain a medical clearance from the patient's physician • Obtain the patient's latest blood test results incl. full blood examination (FBE), liver function test (LFT) • Reduce the recommended BZD dose
Polypharmacy use	• Serious drug interactions • Respiratory depression	• Do NOT prescribe BZD without a prior pharmacy review and a primary care physician consult • Reduce BZD dose in the elderly
Neurological conditions (e.g., depression, treatment with other sedatives)	• Serious drug interactions • Suicidal ideation • Respiratory depression	Do NOT prescribe BZD
Respiratory pathology	• Respiratory depression (higher risk than all other groups)	Do NOT prescribe BZD
Adults aged 65 and over	• Dizziness • Confusion • Dehydration • Falls • Pathologic bone fractures • Respiratory depression	• Obtain a medical clearance from the patient's physician • Reduce dose • Ensure you are ACLS-certified and your clinic staff are BLS-certified
Pregnancy	• Birth defects • Respiratory depression • Neonatal depression	Do NOT prescribe BZD unless cleared by the patient's Ob-Gyn

* All patient groups are at risk of addiction when taking benzodiazepines.

Table 3. Best Practice Recommendations for Anxiolytic Treatment

Obtain a thorough medical and medication history prior to considering prescribing anxiolytics, including baseline vitals and updates at each appointment.

A number of patients are poor historians; contact the patient's physician and pharmacist to clarify medical and medication histories.

For first time users of sedatives, it is advisable to book patients for short appointment as this allows the clinician to assess the patient's coping ability with the chosen sedation technique.

Do not prescribe anxiolytics or pain medications to patients on methadone or buprenorphine therapy as these patients usually have a pain contract in place with their medical provider, usually an addiction specialist with whom prescribing of anxiolytics and pain medications should be coordinated.

Familiarize yourself with anxiolytic contraindications and drug interactions.

Do not prescribe large quantities of anxiolytics; prescribe sufficient quantities for two appointments – this will prevent stockpiling.

Prescribe the minimum recommended/effective anxiolytic dose for the shortest time period: this will reduce adverse effects.

Document the following in the patient's chart:
- time the dose was administered
- minimum effective dose (patient-specific)
- how the patient reacted to, and tolerated, the prescribed dose; this will help guide you for dose adjustment for returning patients

Pre-operative preparation: Before operating on the patient during sedation therapy, ensure the following:
- the patient has a companion who will drive them home: if no companion is present, cancel or reschedule the procedure
- the patient has taken their oral sedative medication as prescribed, the night before and an hour prior to their appointment

Post-operative care and documentation: at the end of the appointment, ensure the following:
- obtain vitals prior to dismissal: BP, heart rate, respiration rate
- document the time the patient was dismissed from the practice
- document the state of patient at dismissal – e.g., patient left in good condition with companion

| **Suggested Reading List**

- American Dental Association. Guidelines for teaching pain control and sedation to dentists and dental students, October 2016. *http://www.ADA.org/~/media/ADA/Education%20and%20Careers/Files/ADA_Sedation_Teaching_Guidelines.pdf?la=en.* Accessed August 3, 2018.

- American Dental Association. 2016 ADA Guidelines for the Use of Sedation and General Anesthesia by Dentists, October 2016. *http://www.ADA.org/~/media/ADA/Education%20and%20Careers/Files/anesthesia_use_guidelines.pdf.* Accessed August 3, 2018.

- American Psychiatric Association. Diagnostic and statistical manual of mental disorders. 5th ed. Text revision. Washington (DC): American Psychiatric Association; 2013.

- American Society of Dentist Anesthesiologists. Sedation. *http://www.asdahq.org/sedation.* Accessed November 1, 2017.

- Chanpong B, Haas DA, Locker D. Need and demand for sedation or general anesthesia in dentistry: a national survey of the Canadian population. Anesth Prog 2005;52:3-11.

- Fuentes D, Gorenstein C, Hu LW. Dental anxiety and trait anxiety: an investigation of their relationship. Br Dent J 2009;206(8):E17.

- Kessler RC, Berglund P, Demler O, et al. Lifetime prevalence and age-of-onset distributions of DSM-IV disorders in the National Comorbidity Survey Replication. Arch Gen Psychiatry 2005;62(6):593–602.

- Moore R. Brødsgaard I, Rosenberg N. The contribution of embarrassment to phobic dental anxiety: a qualitative research study. BMC Psychiatry 2004 Apr 19;4:10.

- Antony MM, Swinson RP. Anxiety disorders and their treatment: a critical review of the evidence-based literature. Ottawa (ON): Health Canada; 1996.

- Milgrom P, Weinstein P. Treating fearful dental patients. Seattle: University of Washington in Seattle, Continuing Dental Education, 1996.

- Rickels K, DeMartinis N, Rynn M, Mandos L. Pharmacologic strategies for discontinuing benzodiazepine treatment. J Clin Psychopharm 1999;19 (suppl 2):12S-16S.

Drug Monograph

The following tables list some anxiolytics that are commonly used in dentistry

NOTE: The sample prescriptions in this handbook represent a general recommendation. Clinicians are responsible to adjust the prescription dose, frequency and length of treatment based on the procedure performed, the medicine prescribed, and the patient conditions such as age, weight, metabolism, liver and renal function.

Anxiolytics are not recommended for use during pregnancy. To achieve drowsiness in pregnant patients prior to a dental procedure, prescribe Diphenhydramine 25mg: Take 2 tablets 30 minutes prior to dental appointment (2 tablets) (Pregnancy Category B).

Diazepam
Tablets: 2 mg, 5 mg
Liquid: 1 mg/mL, 5 mg/mL

ORAL CONDITIONS	• Dental anxiety
SAMPLE PRESCRIPTION	• Take 1 tablet (2 mg) the evening before and 1 tablet (2 mg) one hour before your dental appointment. (2 tablets)
CONTRAINDICATIONS	• BZD allergy (cross-sensitivity with other BZD) • Pregnancy (Category D) • Liver and kidney disease • Acute narrow-angle glaucoma
CAUTIONS	• Increase risk of falls in the elderly due to long-acting active metabolite
MAJOR & SEVERE DRUG INTERACTIONS	• Central Nervous System (CNS) depressants and narcotics: additive CNS depressant effects • Alcohol: additive CNS depressant effects • Antihistamines: additive CNS depressants effects • Oral contraceptive pill: increase in t1/2 and plasma levels of diazepam • Grapefruit/grapefruit juice: may increase levels • Ranitidine: increase in diazepam levels • Anti-fungal drugs: inhibit the hepatic metabolism of diazepam resulting in its elevated serum levels and toxicity
ADVERSE DRUG REACTIONS	Common reactions: • Nausea and vomiting • Dizziness and drowsiness • Lightheadedness and headaches • Ataxia • Falls in the elderly • Poor judgment
PATIENT CONSIDERATIONS	• Pregnancy Category D • Lactation risk category: express milk or use formula up to 48 hours following administration • Pediatric: not recommended • Elderly and ASA III patients: adjust dose • Adjust dose in hepatic disease, and avoid in severe cases • Do not drink alcohol for 2 days prior and 2 days following sedation • Do not drive or operate machinery for 24 hours following sedation
DRUG CONSIDERATIONS	• Onset of action: slow • Peak onset (in hours): 2-3 • Half-life of parent drug (in hours): 3-18 • Active metabolite: no

Triazolam
Tablets: 0.125 mg, 0.25 mg

ORAL CONDITIONS	• Dental anxiety
SAMPLE PRESCRIPTION	• Take 1 tablet (0.25 mg) the evening before and 1 tablet one hour before appointment (2 tablets)
CONTRAINDICATIONS	• BZD allergy (cross-sensitivity with other BZD) • Pregnancy (Category X) • Breast-feeding • Liver and kidney disease • Acute narrow-angle glaucoma • Myasthenia Gravis
CAUTIONS	• Depression: contact the patient's medical practitioner and discuss the suitability of using triazolam
MAJOR & SEVERE DRUG INTERACTIONS	• Central Nervous System (CNS) depressants and narcotics: additive CNS depressant effects • Alcohol: additive CNS depressant effects • Antihistamines: additive CNS depressants effects • Oral contraceptive pill: increase in half life and plasma levels of triazolam • Ranitidine: increase in triazolam levels • Anti-fungal drugs: inhibit the hepatic metabolism of diazepam resulting in its elevated serum levels and toxicity
ADVERSE DRUG REACTIONS	Common reactions: • Nausea and vomiting • Dizziness and drowsiness • Lightheadedness and headaches • Ataxia • Falls in the elderly • Poor judgement
PATIENT CONSIDERATIONS	• Pregnancy Category X • Lactation: express milk or use formula up to 4 hours following administration • Pediatric: not recommended • Elderly and ASA III patients: adjust dose • Adjust dose in hepatic disease, and avoid in severe cases. • Do not drink alcohol for 2 days prior and 2 days following sedation • Do not drive or operate machinery for 24 hours following sedation
DRUG CONSIDERATIONS	• Onset of action: intermediate • Peak onset (in hours): 0.75-2 • Half-life of parent drug (in hours): 1-1.5 • Active metabolite: no

Chapter 6:
Fluorides (Topical and Systemic)

Kathleen Ziegler, PharmD

Overview

Fluoride is a mineral that is found in all natural water sources. Fluoride is the ionic form of the trace element fluorine. Fluorine is commonly found in the environment and reaches water sources by leaching from soil and rocks into groundwater.

The process of caries is multifactorial and, over time, can culminate in localized destruction of hard dental tissues by the weak acids produced by bacterial carbohydrate fermentation. Fluoride remineralizes the calcium hydroxyapatite structure in enamel by forming calcium fluorapatite, which is more resistant to acid attacks. The remineralization effect of fluoride can both reverse the early decay process and create a tooth surface that is more resistant to decay.

Fluoride can be delivered topically and systemically. Topical fluorides strengthen teeth already present in the mouth, making them more decay resistant. Topical fluorides encourage remineralization of enamel, and also inhibit bacterial metabolism, reducing the growth of plaque bacteria. Modes of topical fluoride delivery include toothpastes, gels, mouthrinses, and professionally applied fluoride therapies.

Systemic fluorides are those that are ingested and become incorporated into forming tooth structures. Systemic fluorides can also confer topical protection because fluoride is present in saliva, which continually bathes the teeth. Modes of systemic fluoride delivery include water fluoridation or dietary fluoride supplements in the form of tablets, drops, or lozenges.

1 | Fluorosis

A potential risk of fluoride is the development of fluorosis. Fluorosis of permanent teeth occurs when an excess quantity of fluoride is ingested for a sufficient period while tooth enamel is being mineralized. The level of fluoride intake between the ages of about 15 and 30 months is thought to be most critical for the development of fluorosis of the maxillary central incisors. The mechanisms by which fluoride modifies tooth development are not fully understood, but may result from alterations in protein metabolism disrupting the crystal organization in the developing tooth. Once teeth erupt, they cannot develop enamel fluorosis.

Fluorosis varies in appearance from white striations to stained pitting of enamel and does not affect the function or health of the teeth. Excess fluoride exposure can be minimized by using the recommended amount of toothpaste (Table 1) and by storing toothpaste where young children cannot access it without parental assistance. Parents should supervise their child's use of fluoride toothpaste to avoid overuse or ingestion.

Table 1. ADA Recommendations on Toothpaste Use by Age*	
Age	Amount of Dentifrice
< 3 years	Smear amount of dentifrice
3 to 6 years of age	Pea-sized amount of dentifrice
> 6 years	Regular amount of dentifrice

*See complete guideline at *https://ebd.ADA.org*

2 | Professionally Applied Topical Fluorides

Fluoride Gels, or Foams

Professionally-applied fluorides are more concentrated than self-applied fluorides, and therefore are not needed as frequently. Because these applications are relatively infrequent, generally at 3- to 12-month intervals, fluoride gel poses little risk for dental fluorosis, even among patients younger than six years of age. Routine use of professionally-applied fluoride gel or foam likely provides benefit to persons at high risk for tooth decay, especially those who do not consume fluoridated water and brush daily with fluoride toothpaste.

Because early studies reported that fluoride uptake by dental enamel increased in an acidic environment, fluoride gel is often formulated to be highly acidic (pH of approximately 3.0). Products available in the United States include gels of acidulated phosphate fluoride (1.23% [12,300 ppm] fluoride), as 2% neutral sodium fluoride products (containing 9,000 ppm fluoride), and as gels or foams of sodium fluoride (0.9% [9,040 ppm] fluoride). In a dental office, fluoride gel is generally applied for 1 to 4 minutes, depending on the product used and manufacturer's directions.

Fluoride-Containing Prophylaxis Paste

According to the Centers for Disease Control and Prevention, "Fluoride-containing paste is routinely used during dental prophylaxis (i.e., cleaning). The abrasive paste, which contains 4,000-20,000 ppm fluoride, might restore the concentration of fluoride in the surface layer of enamel removed by polishing, but it is not an adequate substitute for fluoride gel or varnish in treating persons at high risk for dental caries (151). Fluoride paste is not accepted by FDA or ADA as an efficacious way to prevent dental caries." (Recommendations for Using Fluoride to Prevent and Control Dental Caries in the United States (*https://www.cdc.gov/mmwr/preview/mmwrhtml/rr5014a1.htm*).

Fluoride Varnish

Varnishes are available as sodium fluoride (2.26% [22,600 ppm] fluoride) or difluorsilane (0.1% [1,000 ppm] fluoride) preparations. A typical application requires 0.2 to 0.5 mL, resulting in a total fluoride ion application of approximately 5 to 11 mg.

High-concentration fluoride varnish is painted by dental or other health care professionals directly onto the teeth and sets when it comes into contact with saliva. Fluoride varnish is not intended to adhere permanently; this method holds a high concentration of fluoride in a small amount of material in close contact with the teeth for several hours. Reapplying varnishes at regular intervals with at least two applications per year can help effectiveness. Although it is not currently cleared for marketing by the FDA as an anticaries agent, fluoride varnish has been widely used for this purpose in Canada and Europe since the 1970s. Studies conducted in Canada and Europe have reported that fluoride varnish is as effective in managing tooth decay as professionally-applied fluoride gel. In the United States, fluoride varnish is cleared for marketing by the FDA for use as a cavity liner and a root densensitizer, although it has been used "off label" to prevent caries (Recommendations for Using Fluoride to Prevent and Control Dental Caries in the United States (*https://www.cdc.gov/mmwr/preview/mmwrhtml/rr5014a1.htm*).

According to the Centers for Disease Control and Prevention (CDC), there is no published evidence to indicate that professionally-applied fluoride varnish is a risk factor for dental fluorosis, even among children younger than six years of age. Proper application technique reduces the possibility that a patient will swallow varnish during its application and limits the total amount of fluoride swallowed as the varnish wears off the teeth over a period of hours (Recommendations for Using Fluoride to Prevent and Control Dental Caries in the United States (*https://www.cdc.gov/mmwr/preview/mmwrhtml/rr5014a1.htm*).

Silver Diamine Fluoride

Silver diamine fluoride (SDF) referred to 38% SDF is a colorless liquid that at pH 10 is 24.4% to 28.8% (weight/volume) silver and 5.0% to 5.9% fluoride. (Lower concentrations of 12% SDF exist on the market too). The FDA has classified SDF as a Class II medical device and it is cleared for use in the treatment of tooth sensitivity, similar to fluoride varnish, and must be professionally applied. Although some products are commercially available in other countries, currently, Advantage Arrest™ (Elevate Oral Care, L.L.C.) is the only commercially available SDF product for dental use in the United States. There have been reports of the use of SDF in caries arrest and management, although it is not specifically labeled for use for this indication (i.e., "off-label use"). Likely a result of its fluoride content, when applied to a carious lesion, SDF has been shown to lower caries risk of the tooth treated as well as of the adjacent tooth surface. SDF has also shown efficacy in management of root caries in the elderly. It likely has additional applicability as an interim approach for managing problematic caries in individuals currently unable to tolerate more involved dental treatment.

Single application of SDF has been reported to be insufficient for sustained benefit. Its downsides include a reportedly unpleasant metallic taste, potential to irritate gingival and mucosal surfaces, and the characteristic black staining of the carious tooth surfaces to which it is applied.

3 | ADA Clinical Recommendations for Topical Fluorides

In 2013, the ADA Center for Evidence-Based Dentistry and a panel of experts convened by the ADA Council on Scientific Affairs developed clinical recommendations for use of professionally applied or prescription-strength, home-use topical fluorides for caries prevention in patients at high risk of developing caries (See ebd.ada.org for guidelines).

Based on a literature review and consensus, the panel recommended use of the following for caries prevention in patients at elevated risk:

- 2.26% fluoride varnish or 1.23% fluoride (acidulated phosphate fluoride) gel, or a prescription-strength, home-use 0.5% fluoride gel or paste or 0.09% fluoride mouth rinse for patients 6 years or older
- Only 2.26% fluoride varnish was recommended for children younger than 6 years

The strengths of the recommendations for the recommended products varied from "in favor of" to "expert opinion for." The report states that as part of the evidence-based approach to care, these clinical recommendations "should be integrated with the practitioner's professional judgment and the patient's needs and preferences." The panel also determined that patients at low risk of developing caries may receive additional benefit from application of topical fluorides beyond that achieved from their daily use of over-the-counter fluoridated toothpaste and consumption of fluoridated water.

4 | Systemic Fluorides and Suggested Dosing Table

Dietary fluoride supplements can be prescribed for children ages six months to 16 years who are at high risk for caries and whose primary drinking water has a low fluoride concentration. Dosing is based on the natural fluoride concentration of the child's drinking water and the age of the child (Table 2).

Table 2. ADA Recommended Fluoride Supplement Dosage Schedule*			
Age	Fluoride Ion Level in Drinking Water (ppm)		
	<0.3	0.3-0.6	>0.6
Birth-6 months	None	None	None
6 months-3 years	0.25 mg/day	None	None
3-6 years	0.50 mg/day	0.25 mg/day	None
6-16 years	1.0 mg/day	0.50 mg/day	None

** Adapted from: American Academy of Pediatric Dentistry. Guideline on Fluoride Therapy. *http://www.aapd.org/media/Policies_Guidelines/BP_FluorideTherapy.pdf*. Accessed August 3, 2018.

Important considerations when using this dosage schedule include:

- If fluoride level is unknown, drinking water should be tested for fluoride content before supplements are prescribed. For testing of fluoride content, contact the local or state health department.
- All sources of fluoride should be evaluated with a thorough fluoride history.
- Patient exposure to multiple water sources can complicate proper prescribing.
- Ingestion of higher than recommended levels of fluoride by children has been associated with an increased risk of dental fluorosis in developing, unerupted teeth.
- To obtain the benefits from fluoride supplements, long-term compliance on a daily basis is required.
- In 2015, the U.S. Department of Health and Human Services (HHS) has determined 0.7 milligrams of fluoride per liter of water is the optimal fluoride level in drinking water for the prevention of tooth decay.

📖 | **Suggested Reading**

- ADA. Fluoridation Facts: American Dental Association; 2018.
- Centers for Disease and Prevention. Other Fluoride Products. U.S. Department of Health and Human Services. *https://www.cdc.gov/fluoridation/basics/fluoride-products.html*. Accessed. August 3, 2018.
- Horst JA, Ellenikiotis H, Milgrom PL. UCSF Protocol for Caries Arrest Using Silver Diamine Fluoride: Rationale, Indications and Consent. J Calif Dent Assoc 2016;44(1):16-28.
- Recommendations for using fluoride to prevent and control dental caries in the United States. Centers for Disease Control and Prevention. MMWR Recomm Rep 2001;50(Rr-14):1-42.
- Rozier RG, Adair S, Graham F, et al. Evidence-based clinical recommendations on the prescription of dietary fluoride supplements for caries prevention: a report of the American Dental Association Council on Scientific Affairs. J Am Dent Assoc 2010;141(12):1480-9.
- Weyant RJ, Tracy SL, Anselmo TT, et al. Topical fluoride for caries prevention: executive summary of the updated clinical recommendations and supporting systematic review. J Am Dent Assoc 2013;144(11):1279-91.

Drug Monograph

The following tables provide information on prescription fluorides, professionally used fluorides, and over the counter fluorides commonly used in dentistry today.

NOTE: The sample prescriptions in this handbook represent a general recommendation. Clinicians are responsible to adjust the prescription dose, frequency and length of treatment based on the procedure performed, the medicine prescribed, and the patient conditions such as age, weight, metabolism, liver and renal function.

Prescription Systemic Fluorides

Chewable Tablets: 0.25 mg, 0.5 mg, 1 mg
Liquid: 0.125 mg per drop (1 drop = 0.05 mL)
Lozenges: 1 mg

ORAL CONDITIONS	• Prevention of caries
SAMPLE PRESCRIPTION	• Chewable tablets: Chew 1 tablet (1 mg) daily for 30 days (30 tablets) + Refills *Sample prescription is for a patient whose age is between 6 and 16 years old living in an area where water has < 0.3 ppm F ion* *Dosing depends on age of the patient and the local fluoride content of water supply (Refer to Table 2 above for dosing recommendations)*
CONTRAINDICATIONS	• Not indicated if patient lives in an adequately fluoridated area
CAUTIONS	• Do not exceed recommended dosage or fluorosis may occur
MAJOR & SEVERE DRUG INTERACTIONS	• Calcium-containing products and food interfere with absorption of systemic fluorides
ADVERSE DRUG REACTIONS	• Dental fluorosis, if used in excess • If overdoses are consumed (e.g., acute ingestion of 10 to 20 mg of sodium fluoride in children), excessive salivation and gastrointestinal upset can occur; ingestion of larger overdoses (e.g., 500 mg sodium fluoride) can be fatal
PATIENT CONSIDERATIONS	• Excreted in the breast milk • Calcium-containing products and food interfere with absorption of systemic fluorides • Chew tablets or lozenges before swallowing, take at night after brushing teeth • Keep fluoride products away from children
DRUG CONSIDERATIONS	• Absorption: 90% in the stomach; After absorption, 50% of fluoride is deposited in bones and teeth in healthy adults (80% in children); bones and teeth account for 99% of fluoride taken up by the body • Elimination: urine (major); tears and sweat glands (minor)

Professionally-Applied Topical Fluorides

ORAL CONDITIONS	• Prevention of caries
SAMPLE PRESCRIPTION	• Fluoride Solutions, Gels or Foams (0.9% or 1.23% F ion): Use 5 mL (approximately ⅓ of a tray of solution or gel or ¼ of a tray of foam) per arch, following prophylaxis, then apply for 1 to 4 minutes once yearly or more often as needed • Fluoride Varnishes (5% NaF or 1% difluorsilane): Use 0.3 to 0.5 mL of varnish applied to clean, then dry teeth • Fluoride Pastes (0.4% to 2% F ion): Use amount sufficient to polish the teeth
CONTRAINDICATIONS	• Ulcerative gingivitis and stomatitis with fluoride varnishes
CAUTIONS	• Excessive polishing may remove more fluoride from the enamel surface that the prophylaxis paste can replace
MAJOR & SEVERE DRUG INTERACTIONS	• Do not administer other fluoride preparations such as fluoride gels during the same day of fluoride varnish application • The routine use of fluoride tablets should be interrupted for several days after treatment
ADVERSE DRUG REACTIONS	Fluoride Solutions, Gels, or Foams: • Gagging, nausea, vomiting Fluoride Varnishes: • Dyspnea in asthmatic patients • Edematous swelling • Some coloring agents in fluoride gels and solutions can cause allergic reactions (e.g., tartrazine)
PATIENT CONSIDERATIONS	• Do not eat, drink or rinse for 30 minutes, following expectoration of fluoride solution, gel, or foam • Avoid solid foods, alcohol, brushing, and flossing for 4 hours after application of fluoride varnish
DRUG CONSIDERATIONS	None

Self-Applied Topical Fluorides

(Refer to Chapter 12: OTC Products with the ADA Seal of Acceptance
for a complete list of dentifrices and mouthrinses)

ORAL CONDITIONS	• Prevention of caries
SAMPLE PRESCRIPTION	• Brush your teeth twice a day with a fluoride toothpaste *Amount of dentifrice varies per age group (Refer to Table 1)*
CONTRAINDICATIONS	• Use of fluoride rinses in children younger than age 6 years is not recommended • Do not swallow
CAUTIONS	• Allergic reactions to some flavoring agents • Patients with mucositis may report irritation with acidulated formulations
MAJOR & SEVERE DRUG INTERACTIONS	None
ADVERSE DRUG REACTIONS	• Nausea and vomiting may result from inadvertent swallowing • Reversible black staining of pits, fissures, and cervical aspects of teeth can occur with stannous fluoride formulations
PATIENT CONSIDERATIONS	• Following expectoration of fluoride solution or gel, patients should not eat, drink, or rinse for 30 minutes
DRUG CONSIDERATIONS	None

Chapter 7:
Local Anesthetics for Dentistry

Paul A. Moore, DMD, PhD, MPH and Elliot V. Hersh, DMD, MS, PhD

Overview

1 | Chemical Characteristics and Anesthetic Properties

One of the most important elements of pain management in dentistry is the capability to provide effective local anesthesia. The local anesthetic agents available today provide the practitioner multiple options to effectively manage the pain associated with dental procedures.

These agents are extremely safe and fulfill most of the characteristics of an ideal local anesthetic. They all can be administered with minimal tissue irritation, have an extremely low incidence of allergic reactions, while providing rapid onsets and adequate durations of surgical anesthesia.

The clinical characteristics of the local anesthetic agents such as onset times, potency and duration, can be attributed to differences in chemical properties of their molecular structures:

- The more an anesthetic exists in an ionized state, the slower is its onset time. This is the case of ester anesthetics in general. For example, procaine (Novacain), with a pKa of 8.9, is 98% ionized at a normal tissue pH of 7.4 and has a very slow onset.
- The lipid solubility characteristics of a local anesthetic best predict potency. Procaine is one of the least lipid soluble and least potent local anesthetics while bupivacaine is very lipid soluble and one of the most potent
- The protein binding characteristics are a primary determinant of the duration of anesthesia. Lidocaine's short duration and bupivacaine's long duration are due, in part, to their distinctly different protein binding characteristics.

It is thus clear that lipid solubility, ionization and protein binding properties contribute to the clinical characteristics of local anesthetics. However, factors such as the site of injection, inclusion of a vasoconstrictor, concentration and volume of the injected drug, and inherent vasodilatory properties of the anesthetic, also influence the clinical performance of a local anesthetic.

2 | Pharmacological Properties of Amide Local Anesthetics

Because of their superior chemical and anesthetic properties, rarely reported allergenic reactions, and excellent safety profiles, only amide anesthetics are currently formulated into dental cartridges for injection.

Lidocaine Hydrochloride (Formulated as 2% lidocaine with 1:100,000 epinephrine and 2% lidocaine with 1:50,000 epinephrine)

Lidocaine, the first amide anesthetic, was introduced into dental practice in the 1950s and has become one of most popular dental local anesthetics in the United States. Besides having excellent anesthetic efficacy, lidocaine has limited allergenicity.

The 2% lidocaine with 1:100,000 epinephrine is considered the gold standard when evaluating the efficacy and safety of newer anesthetics. The 1:50,000 epinephrine formulation is employed for infiltration injection when additional hemostasis is required.

Mepivacaine Hydrochloride (Formulated as 3% mepivacaine plain and 2% mepivacaine 1:20,000 levonordefrin)

Mepivacaine has an important place in dental anesthesia because it has minimal vasodilating properties and can therefore provide profound local anesthesia without requiring a vasoconstrictor such as epinephrine or levonordefrin. The availability of a 3% formulation not containing a vasoconstrictor is a valuable addition to a dentist's armamentarium.

Prilocaine Hydrochloride (Formulated as 4% prilocaine plain and 4% prilocaine with 1:200,000 epinephrine)

Similar to mepivacaine, prilocaine is not a potent vasodilator and can provide excellent oral anesthesia either with or without a vasoconstrictor. The formulation containing epinephrine has anesthetic characteristics similar to 2% lidocaine 1:100,000 epinephrine. One of prilocaine's metabolic products (toluidine) has been associated with the development of methemoglobinemia.

Articaine Hydrochloride (Formulated as 4% articaine with 1:100,000 epinephrine and 4% articaine with 1:200,000 epinephrine)

The molecular structure of the amide local anesthetic articaine is somewhat unique, containing a thiophene (sulfur-containing) ring. Studies evaluating mandibular block and maxillary infiltration anesthesia, have generally found onset times, duration and anesthetic profundity of articaine formulations to be comparable to 2% lidocaine with 1:100,000 epinephrine.

There is a developing clinical research literature supporting articaine's superior diffusion properties and that anesthesia may be possibly induced following buccal infiltration in the mandible.

Bupivacaine Hydrochloride (Formulated as 0.5% bupivacaine 1:200,000 epinephrine)

The long-acting amide local anesthetics bupivacaine has found an important place in dentists' armamentarium. Bupivacaine is the only long-acting local anesthetic agent formulated in a dental cartridge. When compared to short-acting local anesthetics, bupivacaine's prolonged soft tissue and periosteal anesthesia has been shown to limit post-operative pain. This clinical characteristic is a valuable asset in the overall management of surgical and postoperative pain associated with dental care.

Caution is advised especially in children because of the prolonged anesthesia effects associated with lip biting and trauma.

Clinical trials have shown that bupivacaine, having a pKa of 8.1, has a slightly slower onset time than conventional amide anesthetics.

A combination strategy for managing postoperative pain using a nonsteroidal anti-inflammatory analgesic such as ibuprofen or naproxen, prior to or immediately following surgery in combination with a long-acting anesthetic following surgery, may limit the need for opioid analgesic.

Table 1. Injectable Local Anesthetic Agents*			
Anesthetic Agent	Agent/Formulation	Duration of Pulpal Anesthesia	Pregnancy Category**
Articaine *Brand Names:* Articadent Septocaine Ultracaine Zorcaine	4% articaine/1:100,000 epinephrine	Medium	C
	4% articaine/1:200,000 epinephrine	Medium	C
Bupivacaine *Brand Names:* Marcaine Sensorcaine Vivacaine	0.5% bupivacaine/1:200,000 epinephrine	Long	C
Lidocaine *Brand Names:* Xylocaine Lignospan Alphacaine Octocaine	2% lidocaine/1:100,000 epinephrine	Medium	B
	2% lidocaine/1:50,000 epinephrine	Medium	B
Mepivacaine *Brand Names:* Carbocaine Polocaine Scandonest	3% mepivacaine plain	Short	C
	2% mepivacaine/1:20,000 levonordefrin	Medium	C
Prilocaine *Brand Name:* Citanest	4% prilocaine plain	Short	B
	4% prilocaine/1:200,000 epinephrine	Medium	B

* See the drug monograph for local anesthetic agents at the end of the chapter.
** Drugs that have Pregnancy Category Rating of "C" should be used with caution during pregnancy.

3 | Adverse Reactions Associated with Local Anesthetics

Methemoglobinemia

There are two local anesthetic agents used in dentistry that reportedly induce methemoglobinemia. The first agent is the topical local anesthetic benzocaine and the second agent is the injectable (and topical) local anesthetic prilocaine. The mechanism of action is that both of these anesthetics oxidize hemoglobin to methemoglobin. As the level of methemoglobin continues to increase in the blood, cyanosis develops and additional symptoms appear with the potential for progression to unconsciousness and death. This phenomena invariably occurs with excessive dose of either agent. Fortunately, methemoglobinemia treatments using methylene blue are generally effective.

Systemic Toxicity Reactions Due to Excessive Local Anesthetic

When excessive doses of any of these local anesthetics are administered, excitatory central nervous system (CNS) reactions, such as tremors, muscle twitching, shivering and clonic-tonic convulsions have been reported. These initial excitatory reactions are thought to be due to a selective blockade of small inhibitory neurons within the limbic system of the CNS. Whether this initial excitatory reaction is apparent or not, a generalized CNS depression with symptoms of sedation, drowsiness, lethargy and life-threatening respiratory depression follows if blood concentrations of the local anesthetic agent continue to rise. Severe bradycardia may also occur due to the ability of local anesthetics to block sodium channels in the heart. Compliance with local anesthetic dosing guidelines is the first and most important strategy for preventing this adverse event. Dosing calculations used to avoid systemic reactions to local anesthetics are dependent on the agent administered and the patient's body weight (Table 2).

Toxicity Reactions Due to Excessive Vasoconstrictors

Epinephrine and levonordefrin are the two vasoconstrictors formulated with local anesthetic agents in dental cartridges. The use of a vasoconstrictor can improve the safety of the formulation by slowing the systemic absorption of the local anesthetic and decrease the peak blood levels of the anesthetic. There is minimal stimulation of the cardiovascular system following submucosal injection of one or two cartridges of anesthetic containing epinephrine or levonordefrin. However, when excessive amounts of these vasoconstrictors are administered, or when inadvertently administered intravascularly, cardiovascular stimulation, with clinically significant increases in blood pressure and heart rate, can occur. Using anesthetic formulations containing no or limited amounts of vasoconstrictors, using a slow injection technique, and aspirating carefully and repeatedly are common recommendations to prevent rapid systemic absorption of epinephrine and levonordefrin.

Although vasoconstrictors are rarely contraindicated, the potential stimulation of the cardiovascular system following intravascular injections should guide the dental practitioners to avoid vasoconstrictor-containing formulations in cardiovascularly compromised populations if possible. A common recommendation, when a vasoconstrictor is required for a dental treatment and when there is a medical history that suggests a need for caution, is to limit the dose of epinephrine to 0.04 mg (See Section 2 for information specific to children). This can be achieved by limiting the total anesthetics used to: one cartridge of an anesthetic containing 1:50,000 epinephrine, two cartridges of an anesthetic containing 1:100,000 epinephrine, or four cartridges of an anesthetic containing 1:200,000 epinephrine.

Table 2. Maximum Recommended Dosages of Injectable Local Anesthetics

Agents/ Formulation*	Local Anesthetic		Epi/Levo mg/cart.‡	MRD§		Max Cart. (number)	
	mg/ mL	mg/ cart.†		Adult (mg)	mg/lbs§	Adult	25 lb. Child
2% Lidocaine, 1:100,000 epi	20	36	0.018	500	3.3	11.1¶	2.3
2% Lidocaine, 1:50,000 epi	20	36	0.036	500	3.3	5.55¶	2.3
4% Articaine, 1:100,000 epi	40	72	0.018	500	3.3	6.9	1.1
4% Articaine, 1:200,000 epi	40	72	0.009	500	3.3	6.9	1.1
3% Mepivacaine	30	54	—	400	2.6	7.4	1.2
2% Mepivacaine, 1:20,000 levo	20	36	0.09	400	2.6	11.1	1.8
4% Prilocaine	40	72	—	600	4.0	8.3	1.4
4% Prilocaine, 1:200,000 epi	40	72	0.009	600	4.0	8.3	1.4
0.5% Bupivacaine, 1:200,000 epi	5	9	0.009	90	0.6	10.0	NR

* epi = epinephrine; levo = levonordefrin
† The volume of a dental cartridge is approximated to 1.8 mL
‡ 1:100,000 epi = 0.01 mg/mL; A 1.8 mL cartridge contains 0.018 mg epi
§ Maximum Recommended Dose (MRD); 1.0 kg = 2.2 lbs; 70 kg adult = 150 lbs
¶ Maximum Recommended Dose (MRD) for epinephrine for a healthy adult is 0.2 mg. The maximum number of cartridges for an adult receiving 2% lidocaine 1:100,000 or 1:50,000 epinephrine are based on the 0.2 mg maximum for epinephrine in these formulations.

4 | Topical Anesthetics for Dentistry

Professional application of topical local anesthetics is a valuable addition to a dentist's pain control armamentarium, providing surface anesthesia that can mitigate the discomfort of anesthetic needle insertion as well as pain from soft tissue lesions, minor gingival and periodontal procedures and possibly small biopsies. When applied in metered amounts to oral mucosa, topical anesthetics have limited absorption and reports of adverse reactions are rare and usually limited to localized allergic reactions.

Table 3. Topical Local Anesthesia

Anesthetic Agent	Topical Formulations	Primary Indications
Lidocaine *Brand name:* Lidocaine Ointment	spray, gel, or ointment	Pre-injection anesthesia
Benzocaine *Brand names:* HurriCaine Topicale Topex	spray, gel, or ointment	Pre-injection anesthesia, toothache, apthous ulcers
Butamben//Benzocaine/ Tetracaine *Brand name:* Cetacaine*	liquid and gel	Periodontal scaling and root planing Suppression of gag reflex
Prilocaine/Lidocaine combination *Brand name:* Oraqix*	EMLA solution	Periodontal Scaling and Root Planing

* See the drug monograph for Cetacaine and Oraqix at the end of the chapter.

📖 | Suggested Reading

- Pharmacology and Therapeutics for Dentistry, 7th edition. Frank Dowd, Bart Johnson, and Angelo Mariotti Editors. Elsevier St Louis, 2017.
- Guay, J., Methemoglobinemia Related to Local Anesthetics: A Summary of 242 Episodes. Anesthesia and Analgesia, 2009. 108(3): p. 837-845
- Moore PA and Haas DA. Paresthesias in Dentistry. Dent Clin North Am 2010;54:715-730.
- Robertson D, Nusstein J, Reader A, Beck M, McCartney M. The anesthetic efficacy of articaine in buccal infiltration of mandibular posterior teeth. J Am Dent Assoc. 2007 Aug;138(8):1104-1112.
- Hersh EV, Moore PA, Pappas AS, Goodson JM. Rutherford B, Rogy, S, Navalta LA, Yageila, and the Soft Tissue Anesthesia Recovery Group. Reversal of soft tissue local anesthesia with phentolamine mesylate in adolescents and adults. J Am Dent Assoc 2008;139:1080-1093.
- Hersh EV, Lindemeyer R, Berg JH, Casamassimo PS, Chin J, Marberger A, Lin BP, Hutcheson MC, Moore PA, Group PS. Phase Four, Randomized, Double-Blinded, Controlled Trial of Phentolamine Mesylate in Two- to Five-year-old Dental Patients. Pediatr Dent. 2017;39(1):39-45.
- Goodson JM and Moore PA: Life-threatening reactions following pedodontic sedation: an assessment of narcotic, local anesthetic and antiemetic drug interaction. J Am Dent Assoc 1983;107:239-45.
- Meechan JG. Intra-oral topical anaesthetics: a review. J Dentistry 2000;28:3-14

Drug Monograph

The following tables list some of the most commonly used anesthetics in dentistry.

Injectable Amide Local Anesthetics
(lidocaine, mepivacaine, prilocaine, articaine, or bupivacaine)

 ORAL CONDITIONS	• Infiltration anesthesia • Nerve block Anesthesia
 FORMULATION & DOSAGE	• Varies depending on the amide formulation used: For lidocaine, mepivacaine, prilocaine, articaine, or bupivacaine, refer to Table 1 for formulation, and refer to Table 2 for dosage
 CONTRAINDICATIONS	• Allergy to amide local anesthetics • Hypersensitivity to any of the components including sulfites
 CAUTIONS	• Avoid intravascular injections by aspiration
 MAJOR & SEVERE DRUG INTERACTIONS	• Drug interaction with the epinephrine component include propranolol, tricyclic antidepressants, MAOIs and phenothiazides • Drug interaction with the local anesthetic component include other CNS depressants
 ADVERSE DRUG REACTIONS	Common reactions: • Injection site tenderness and edema following anesthesia • Vasovagal reactions are common reactions to local anesthetic injections Less common reactions: • Methemoglobinemia • Paresthesias • Asthmatic response to sulfite antioxidants
 PATIENT CONSIDERATIONS	• Pregnancy Category B or C refer to Table 1 on page 61 • Reduce dose of local anesthetic solutions with medically compromised patients • Minimize or avoid epinephrine with patients having cardiac disease history • Resuscitation equipment and drugs should always be available
 DRUG CONSIDERATIONS	None

Tetracaine and Oxymetazoline Nasal Spray
(Kovanaze®)

ORAL CONDITIONS	• Regional anesthesia for restorations on adult teeth 4-13 and primary teeth A-J
FORMULATION & DOSAGE	• Pre-filled, single-use, intranasal sprayer containing a clear 0.2 mL aqueous solution containing tetracaine HCl 30 mg/mL and oxymetazoline HCl 0.5 mg/mL - One spray contains tetracaine 6 mg and oxymetazoline 0.1 mg (formulated at a pH of 6.0 ± 1.0) - Maximum dose in adults: 3 intranasal sprays - Maximum dose in children weighing >40 kg: 2 sprays
CONTRAINDICATIONS	• Allergy to tetracaine, benzyl alcohol, p- aminobenzoic acid (PABA), oxymetazoline • Children under 3 years of age or weighing less that 40 kg • Patients with history of epistaxis
CAUTIONS	• Patient with hypertension • Patient with thyroid disease
MAJOR & SEVERE DRUG INTERACTIONS	• Drug interaction with oxymetazoline include propranolol, MAOIs, tricyclic antidepressants, and phenothiazides • Drug interaction with local anesthetic include other CNS depressants
 **ADVERSE DRUG REACTIONS**	Common reactions: • Rhinorrhea, nasal congestion, transient headache and lacrimation • Elevated blood pressure • Oropharyngeal pain, lacrimation Less common reactions: • Methemoglobinemia • Elevation in blood pressure
PATIENT CONSIDERATIONS	• Pregnancy Category: insufficient evidence to inform risk • Avoid the use of other nasal products for 24 hours • Patients may not experience soft tissue of lips and cheeks
DRUG CONSIDERATIONS	None

Reversal of Soft Tissue Anesthesia

Phentolamine Mesylate
(OraVerse®)

ORAL CONDITIONS	· Reversal of soft tissue anesthesia following dental anesthesia
FORMULATION & DOSAGE	· Phentolamine Mesylate 0.4 mg per 1.7 mL cartridge - Range of dose is 0.1 to 0.8 mg - Dosing is dependent on number of cartridges of local anesthetic
CONTRAINDICATIONS	· Children under 3 years of age or weighing less than 15 kg
CAUTIONS	None
MAJOR & SEVERE DRUG INTERACTIONS	None
ADVERSE DRUG REACTIONS	· Post-procedural pain due to lack of local anesthesia · Acute and prolonged hypotension
PATIENT CONSIDERATIONS	· Pregnancy Category C
DRUG CONSIDERATIONS	· Recovery of normal sensation decreased by 55% following mandibular anesthesia · Recovery of normal sensation decreased by 62% following maxillary anesthesia

Lidocaine/Prilocaine
(Oraqix®)

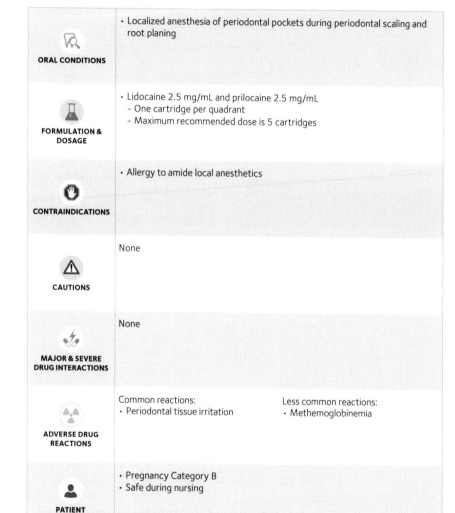

ORAL CONDITIONS	• Localized anesthesia of periodontal pockets during periodontal scaling and root planing

FORMULATION & DOSAGE	• Lidocaine 2.5 mg/mL and prilocaine 2.5 mg/mL
	  - One cartridge per quadrant
	  - Maximum recommended dose is 5 cartridges

CONTRAINDICATIONS	• Allergy to amide local anesthetics
CAUTIONS	None
MAJOR & SEVERE DRUG INTERACTIONS	None
ADVERSE DRUG REACTIONS	Common reactions: • Periodontal tissue irritation Less common reactions: • Methemoglobinemia
PATIENT CONSIDERATIONS	• Pregnancy Category B • Safe during nursing
DRUG CONSIDERATIONS	• Onset time: 1 minute • Duration: 20 minutes

Tetracaine/Benzocaine/Butaben
(Cetacaine®)*

ORAL CONDITIONS	• Localized anesthesia of periodontal pockets during periodontal scaling and root planing • Spray indicated for gag reflex suppresion

FORMULATION & DOSAGE	• Tetracaine HCl 2.0 mg/mL, Benzocaine 14 mg/mL, Butaben 2.0 mg/mL (Gel Liquid and Spray)
	  – Periodontal application of 0.2 mL
	  – Maximum recommended dose is 0.4 mL
	  – Spray application for 1 second
	  – Maximum spray of 2 seconds (est. benzocaine 56 mg, tetracaine 8 mg, butaben 8 mg)

CONTRAINDICATIONS	• Allergy to tetracaine, benzocaine, butaben or similar local anesthetics • Patients with cholinesterase deficiencies
CAUTIONS	None
MAJOR & SEVERE DRUG INTERACTIONS	None
ADVERSE DRUG REACTIONS	Common reactions: • Tissue Irritation and hypersensitivity Less common reactions: • Methemoglobinemia
PATIENT CONSIDERATIONS	• Pregnancy Category: unknown • Avoid during nursing • Not for injection
DRUG CONSIDERATIONS	• Onset time: 0.5-1 minute • Duration: 30 minutes

* New spray formulation in 2020 expected to be devoid of butaben and chloroflurocarbon propellant. The reformulated product will be administered from a metered canister.

Chapter 8:
Oral Lesions and Corticosteroids

Elias Mikael Chatah, DMD, BPharm, MS

NOTE: The pharmacologic management suggestions and sample prescriptions in this handbook represent a general recommendation. Clinicians are responsible to adjust the prescription dose, frequency and length of treatment based on the procedure performed, the medicine prescribed, and the patient conditions such as age, weight, metabolism, liver and renal function.

Overview

Steroids, often referred to as corticosteroids, are hormones produced by the adrenal cortex, the outer part of the adrenal gland. The hormone cortisol is the principal corticosteroid. Cortisol secretion is regulated via the hypothalamic–pituitary–adrenal axis (HPA axis) and by the circadian rhythm. It plays a role in carbohydrate, protein, lipid and nucleic acid metabolism. In addition, cortisol is the main hormone involved in the human stress response with levels being highest in the early morning. Synthetic steroids (i.e., hydrocortisone) are derivatives of cortisol. Synthetic steroids can be used in dentistry topically or systemically as a palliative measure to relieve pain, inflammation or edema.

1 | Oral Lesions: Etiology and Treatment

Topical steroids are not curative but rather palliative. Topical steroid may reduce the severity of oral lesions, reducing pain and improving patient function and quality of life. Topical steroids should be considered the first course of treatment.

Table 1. Aphthous Stomatitis (also known as canker sores)	
Etiology	• Common oral condition, esp. in young adults • Familial tendency • May be caused by stress, physical or chemical trauma, food sensitivity and infection • May be associated with use of NSAIDs
Treatment Rationale	• Most ulcers heal spontaneously in 10-14 days • Inflammation reduction • Pain relief

Suggested Pharmacologic Management	• Rx. Triamcinolone 0.1% in Orabase
	  – Sig: apply to dried ulcer 2-4 times daily until healed
	• Rx. Dexamethasone elixir, 0.5 mg per 5 mL
	  – Sig: rinse with 5 mL for 2 minutes four times daily and spit out. *Discontinue when lesions become asymptomatic*
	• Rx. Tetracycline 250 mg/5 mL syrup
	  – Sig: 5 mL "swish and spit" four times daily for 4-5 days
	• Viscous lidocaine, 2% used to relieve pain

Table 2. Erythema Multiforme (EM)	
Etiology	• Autoimmune disorder • Severe form is called Stevens Johnson syndrome or Erythema Multiforme Major • Allergic reaction to antibiotics, e.g., penicillin • Post-herpetic infection
Treatment Rationale	• Inflammation reduction (systemic steroid therapy) • Following a thorough medical history, if a link to viral infections is established 48 hours following experiencing the symptoms (rash), suppressive antiviral therapy should be considered; due to interference of systemic steroids with the immune system. This approach, if used, should be initiated **prior** to steroid therapy. The goal of antiviral therapy is to shorten the clinical course of EM, prevent further complications and prevent recurrences and the development of latent viral infections and transmission

Suggested Pharmacologic Management	• Rx: Prednisone 10 mg tablets
	  – Sig: take SIX tablets in the morning after breakfast then decrease dose by ONE tablet every other day. (Disp. 42 tablets)
	  Do NOT use for more than 14 days; if lesions do not resolve following 14 days of therapy, patient should contact primary physician
	• Rx.: Valacyclovir 500 mg tablets
	  – Sig: take one tablet twice daily (Disp. 20 tablets)
	• Rx.: Acyclovir 400 mg tablets
	  – Sig: take one tablet twice daily (Disp. 20 tablets)

Table 3. Lichen Planus

Etiology	• Autoimmune disorder • May be caused by stress, drug hypersensitivity or allergen exposure
Treatment Rationale	• Pain relief • Inflammation reduction (Topical steroid application is preferred) • Expect *Candida* overgrowth to occur and treat accordingly; monitor the patient for opportunistic oral infections including candidosis – consider prophylactic antifungal therapy in certain patients, the elderly and denture wearers

Suggested Pharmacologic Management	• Rx.: Fluocinonide Gel 0.05% mixed with equal parts plain Benzocaine 20%
	  – Sig.: Apply to oral lesions 3-4 times daily using a cotton tip applicator (Disp.: 30 g tube)
	    Discontinue when symptoms disappear. If symptoms persist for more than 2 weeks, patient should contact primary physician.
	• Rx.: Dexamethasone Elixir 0.5 mg/5 mL
	  – Sig.: swish with 5 mL (1 tsp) for 2 minutes four times per day then spit out (Disp.: 100 mL)
	    Discontinue when symptoms disappear. If symptoms persist for more than 2 weeks, patient should contact primary physician.

Table 4. Mucous Membranes Pemphigoid (MMP) and Pemphigus Vulgaris (PV)

Etiology	• Autoimmune disorder with antibodies
Treatment Rationale	• Management requires a physician and a dental professional • Control and reduction of the symptoms with systemic corticosteroids, topical steroids and immunomodulators (Tacrolimus has been proven to aid in the control of oral lesions) • Topical steroids usually used as adjunct to oral therapy but can be used as monotherapy in patients with limited oral disease

Suggested Pharmacologic Management	Topical steroid therapy (as for Lichen Planus but part of a larger treatment plan):
	• Rx.: Fluocinonide Gel 0.05% mixed with equal parts plain Benzocaine 20% (consider using a custom tray)
	  – Sig.: Apply to oral lesions 3-4 times daily using a cotton tip applicator (Disp.: 30 g tube)
	    Discontinue when symptoms disappear. If symptoms persist for more than 2 weeks, contact your doctor
	• Rx.: Dexamethasone elixir 0.5 mg/5 mL
	  – Sig.: swish with 5 mL (1 tsp) for 2 minutes four times per day then spit out. (Disp.: 100 mL)
	    Discontinue when symptoms disappear. If symptoms persist for more than 2 weeks, patient should contact primary physician

2 | Oral Lesions: Size and Location

Current dosage forms of topical steroids include creams, gels, powders, lotions, oils, ointments, solutions and sprays. Of interest to the dental clinician are ointments, such as fluocinonide and triamcinolone, due to their carrier being suitable for use in the oral cavity; creams are indicated for dermatologic conditions and are best avoided intra-orally.

Treatment success is related to the location and accessibility of the lesion, and patient compliance:

Lesions Accessible to the Patient

To facilitate adhesion to the oral lesions, which improves contact time and outcome, the clinician should direct the pharmacist to compound topical steroids with equal parts plain Orabase which contains 20% benzocaine in an alcohol-free paste.

Instruct the patient to apply the ointment as follows:

1. Rinse oral cavity with salt water (1 tsp salt in one cup of water).
2. Wash hands prior to applying ointment.
3. Apply ointment to oral lesions 3-4 times daily using a cotton tip applicator.

Lesions Confined to the Gingival Tissue

The clinician can fabricate custom-fitted trays to be filled with the compound described above.

Instruct the patient to apply the ointment as follows:

1. Brush teeth prior to applying medication.
2. Rinse oral cavity with salt water (1 tsp salt in one cup of water).
3. Wash hands prior to applying ointment.
4. Gently insert tray and keep in oral cavity for 15 minutes then remove and do not rinse.
5. Repeat the above steps three times (up to 4 doses per 24 hours).

Lesions that are numerous or inaccessible to the patient

Topical treatment is perhaps not the best option for these lesions. The clinician should consider an elixir (oral rinse) such as dexamethasone elixir (0.5 mg/5 mL).

Instruct the patient to use the elixir as follows:

1. Rinse oral cavity with salt water (1 tsp salt in one cup of water).
2. Rinse with elixir for 3-4 minutes four times daily then expectorate.

Multiple elixirs exist, often referred to as "Magic Mouthwash" combinations. Without any conclusive scientific study on this matter, these compounded elixirs are recommended by many experts in the field. The majority of formulations contains four or more ingredients including:

- an antibiotic for reducing oral bacterial load
- an antihistamine and 2% viscous lidocaine for local anesthesia and pain relief
- an antifungal for reducing the growth of oral fungi
- an oral steroid for reducing local inflammation
- an antacid such as Maalox or Mylanta to act as a barrier and coating for the ingredients.

The combination is related to the lesion diagnosis. The following is an example of a Magic Mouthwash for the treatment of oral mucositis *(adapted from Clarkson JE, Worthington HV, Eden OB. Interventions for treating oral mucositis for patients with cancer receiving treatment. Cochrane Database Syst Rev 2007;(2):CD001973).*

Rx: Mix the following ingredients:

- Viscous lidocaine 2%   80 mL
- Mylanta   80 mL
- Diphenhydramine 12.5 mg/5 mL   80 mL
- Nystatin suspension   80 mL
- Prednisolone 15 mg/5 mL   80 mL
- Distilled water   80 mL

Sig: Swish, gargle, and spit 5 mL to 10 mL every 6 hours as needed. May be swallowed if esophageal involvement.

Keep refrigerated.

3 | Topical Steroids: Classes and Potency

When used appropriately in the oral cavity for a maximum of two weeks, topical steroids are poorly absorbed into the systemic circulation and do not suppress the hypothalamic pituitary adrenal (HPA) axis; the exception is the ultra-potent topical steroid clobetasol, which increases the risk of HPA axis suppression when used for two or more weeks since it is readily absorbed through the oral mucosa and into the systemic circulation.

Factors that increase the risk of systemic absorption include the strength of the steroid, duration of application, body surface area being treated, the integrity of the mucosa and degree of inflammation, and the amount being used. In most cases, HPA axis suppression resolves upon ceasing use of the steroid.

In addition, used for longer than two weeks, topical steroids can result in mucosal atrophy (similar to skin thinning) and secondary candidiasis. As such, patients being treated for conditions that require longer treatment periods such as lichen planus and pemphigoid/pemphigus conditions should be instructed to taper topical steroid application to alternate day application once the condition has improved. Patients should be instructed to apply a "smear" if using an applicator or a custom tray.

Based on their potency, topical steroids can be classified as ultra, high, medium or low.

Table 5. Topical Steroids Potency*		
Potency	Steroid Class (I–VII)	Steroid
Ultra	I	• Clobetasol propionate cream (0.05%) • Diflorasone diacetate ointment (0.05%)
High	II	• Amcinonide ointment (0.1%) • Betamethasone dipropionate ointment (0.05%) • Desoximetasone (cream or ointment) (0.025%) • Fluocinonide (cream, ointment, or gel) (0.05%) • Halcinonide cream (0.1%)
Medium	III–V	Class III: • Betamethasone dipropionate cream (0.05%) • Betamethasone valerate ointment (0.1%) • Diflorasone diacetate cream (0.05%) • Triamcinolone acetonide ointment (0.1%) Class IV: • Desoximetasone cream (0.05%) • Fluocinonide acetonide ointment (0.025%) • Hydrocortisone valerate ointment (0.2%) • Triamcinolone acetonide cream (0.1%) Class V: • Betamethasone dipropionate lotion (0.02%) • Betamethasone valerate cream (0.1%) • Fluocinonide acetonide cream (0.025%) • Hydrocortisone butyrate cream (0.1%) • Hydrocortisone valerate cream (0.2%) • Triamcinolone acetonide lotion (0.1%)
Low	VI–VII	Class VI: • Betamethasone valerate lotion (0.05%) • Desonide cream (0.05%) • Fluocinolone acetonide solution (0.01%) Class VII: • Dexamethasone sodium phosphate cream (0.1%) • Hydrocortisone acetate cream (1%) • Methylprednisolone acetate cream (0.25%)

* See the drug monograph for Dexamethasone at the end of the chapter.

4 | Systemic Steroids: Oro-Dental Indications

The use of systemic steroids in dentistry rarely exceeds four weeks. Regular administration of systemic steroids that continues beyond four weeks is considered long-term treatment and is not typically used in dentistry. Long-term use of steroids by patients should not be ceased without consultation with the prescribing physician as this can result in suppression of the HPA axis, which can result in life-threatening complications. In addition, adverse effects of long-term high dose corticosteroids include bone loss, which may negatively impact dental implant osseointegration. This results from reduced bone formation, increased bone resorption (bone turnover) and osteoporosis long-term. The clinician should make an evidence-based decision as to the suitability of implants in patients on long-term steroid use.

Oro-dental effects of systemic steroid use can include:

- delayed mucosal healing
- increased risk of periodontal infection as a result of the anti-inflammatory activity and reduced immune function

Only pain-producing dental and surgical procedures call for systemic glucocorticoid supplementation or replacement; examples include oral surgery, root canals, pain-producing periodontal scaling (large defects), biopsy, implant placement and bone grafting. Oral examinations and radiographs do not require supplementation.

Alternate day systemic glucocorticoid therapy is common. Patients taking alternate day steroid therapy do not require steroid supplementation prior to dental treatment as this alternate therapy is less suppressive to the HPA axis relative to daily therapy: it is recommended that dental treatment be performed on the day the patient is not taking their steroid dose.

Given that in stressful situations the body produces 250-300 mg of cortisol, the literature recommends supplementation with the equivalent of 300 mg of hydrocortisone or 75 mg of prednisone, taken the morning of the dental procedure. However, the clinician must tailor the dose to the anticipated stress and an anti-anxiety pre-medication should be considered. The clinician is advised to consult with the patient's physician prior to supplementing with long term systemic glucocorticoids therapy. In addition to supplementation, the clinician should use long-acting anesthesia.

When operating on patients who were given supplemental steroids, the clinician is advised to monitor the patient's vital signs and overall well-being throughout treatment.

📖 | **Suggested Reading**

- Alexander RE, Throndson RR. A review of perioperative corticosteroid use in dentoalveolar surgery. Oral Surg Oral Med Oral Pathol Oral Radiol Endod 2000;90(4):406-15.

- Fuller P, Young M. Mechanisms of Mineralocorticoid Action. Hypertension. *https:// www.ahajournals.org/doi/10.1161/01.HYP.0000193502.77417.17?url_ver=Z39.88- 2003&rfr_id=ori:rid:crossref.org&rfr_dat=cr_pub%3dpubmed*. Accessed August 28, 2018.

- Guyton AC, Hall JE. Medical physiology. 10th ed. Philadelphia: W.B. Saunders; 2000.

- Neiman L. Pharmcologic Use of Glucocorticoids. *http://www.uptodate.com/ contents/pharmacologic-use-of-glucocorticoids*. Accessed August 3, 2018.

- Velden V H. Glucocorticoids: Mechanisms of Action and Anti-inflammatory Potential in Asthma, Mediators of Inflammation. U.S. National Library of Medicine. *http:// www.ncbi.nlm.nih.gov/pmc/articles/PMC1781857*. Accessed August 3, 2018.

Drug Monograph

The following table lists an example of a commonly used corticosteroid in dentistry today.

NOTE: The sample prescriptions in this handbook represent a general recommendation. Clinicians are responsible to adjust the prescription dose, frequency and length of treatment based on the procedure performed, the medicine prescribed, and the patient conditions such as age, weight, metabolism, liver and renal function.

Dexamethasone
Tablets 0.5 mg, 0.75 mg, 1 mg, 1.5 mg, 4 mg, 6 mg
Liquid: 0.5mg/5 mL, 1 mg/1 mL

 ORAL CONDITIONS	· Prevention of swelling and edema from oral surgery
 SAMPLE PRESCRIPTION	· Take 2 tablets (2x 4 mg) before surgery then take 1 tablet (4 mg) the day of surgery (3 tablets)
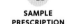 **CONTRAINDICATIONS**	· Hypersensitivity to steroids · Cerebral malaria · Systemic fungal infection · Patients planning to receive live or attenuated vaccines while on corticosteroids therapy
 CAUTIONS	· Diabetes　　　　　　　　　　· Peptic ulceration · Congestive heart failure　　　· Previous steroid myopathy · Epilepsy and other seizure disorders　· Recent myocardial infarction · Glaucoma　　　　　　　　· Renal insufficiency/failure · Hypertension　　　　　　· Tuberculosis · Hypothyroidism　　　　　· Steroid-induced psychoses · Liver failure　　　　　　　· Systemic infections · Osteoporosis
 MAJOR & SEVERE DRUG INTERACTIONS	· This drug ↑ the concentration of NSAIDs and increases the risk of GI ulceration (peptic) · This drug ↓ effect of: 　- Live vaccines such as BCG, cholera, typhoid 　- Inactivated vaccines 　- Cholesterol lowering drugs such as Statins 　- Antidiabetic including insulin 　- GERD drugs such as proton pump inhibitors 　- Anticoagulants and antiplatelet such as warfarin and aspirin · The following family of medications ↓ the effect of this drug: 　- Antacids decrease dexamethasone absorption 　- CYP450 inducers such as phenytoin, rifampicin, St John's wort · The following family of medications ↑ the effect of this drug: 　- CYP450 inhibitors such as clarithromycin, azithromycin, erythromycin, ketoconazole 　- Estrogen replacement therapies
 ADVERSE DRUG REACTIONS	Large doses taken for four weeks or less are likely to result in: Common reactions:　　　　　　Less common reactions: · insomnia and sleep disturbances　· severe infection 　which can result in tiredness　· psychosis, confusion, delirium and · food craving and increased appetite　depression 　resulting in transient weight gain　· cardiovascular problems · mood swings and changes in energy　· gastrointestinal pain and peptic ulceration 　levels　　　　　　　　　　· changes in glucose levels
 PATIENT CONSIDERATIONS	· Pregnancy Category C · Lactation: excreted in milk · Patients with renal insufficiency: consult with PCP · Patients with liver failure; consult with PCP · Need to limit blood pressure-raising foods including salt, licorice etc. · Take with food and during the day, preferably prior to midday as this drug interferes with sleep · Delays male puberty; disrupts reproductive functions via hypothalamic-pituitary-gonadal axis alterations when taken in high doses and for a long period of time
 DRUG CONSIDERATIONS	· Peak plasma concentrations: 1 hr · Plasma protein binding is less than for others corticosteroids · Penetrates tissue and cerebrospinal fluid · Half-life: approx. 190 minutes · Elimination: metabolism and renal excretion

See how dexamethasone compares to other corticosteroids available on the market. Based on their potency, systemic glucocorticoids can be classified as short, intermediate or long-acting.

Table 6. Systemic Glucocorticoid Potency		
	Glucocorticoid Potency	Plasma Half-life (in minutes)
Short-Acting, Low Potency		
Cortisol	1	90
Cortisone	0.8	80–118
Intermediate Potency		
Prednisone	4	60
Prednisolone	4	115–200
Triamcinolone	5	30
Methylprednisolone	5	180
Long-Acting, High Potency		
Dexamethasone	25–50	200
Betamethasone	25–50	300

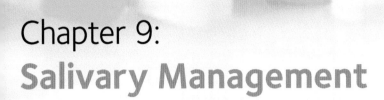

Chapter 9:
Salivary Management

Jay Elkareh, PharmD, PhD

Overview

1 | Hyposalivation

Saliva is a multifunctional substance produced by the body, rich in minerals and salivary proteins. Saliva keeps the oral pH between 6 and 7, and it plays a vital role in protecting the health of the soft and hard oral tissues, assisting in functions such as taste, mastication, and deglutition. Hyposalivation can put patients at risk of bacterial, fungal and viral infections. The loss of lubrication and mucosal integrity exposes patients to oral malaise, pain from inflammation and ulceration.

Hyposalivation is an objective, measurable decrease in saliva secretion, while xerostomia is a subjective sensation of dry mouth experienced by the patient that can occur with or without diminished salivary flow. Normal, unstimulated, salivary secretory rate varies from 0.3 to 0.4 mL/min. In hyposalivation, the unstimulated flow rate falls below 0.1 mL/min. Treatments used for xerostomia vary from over-the-counter products to prescription medications. The three major causes of xerostomia are medication-induced hyposalivation, radiation-induced hyposalivation, and condition-induced hyposalivation.

2 | Medication-Induced Hyposalivation

In general, the most common types of medications causing salivary dysfunction have anticholinergic effects. At present, more than 500 medications possess some kind of anticholinergic properties. Some of them are among the most prescribed medications, and many of them are available over the counter.

Below are some classes of medications that can cause xerostomia, organized by therapeutic class:

- Cardiovascular system:
  - Antiarrhythmic agents, such as digoxin, disopyramide
  - Antihypertensive drugs, such as clonidine, methyldopa
  - Beta Blockers, such as atenolol, timolol, metoprolol
  - Calcium Channel Blockers, such as diltiazem, verapamil
  - Diuretics, such as furosemide, bumetanide

- Central nervous system:
  - Amphetamines, such as dextroamphetamine, methamphetamine
  - Antianxiolytics, such as alprazolam, clonazepam
  - Antidepressants, such as amitriptyline, bupropion, paroxetine, sertraline, fluoxetine, citalopram
  - Antimigraine drugs, such as diergotamine, sumatriptan
  - Antipsychotics, such as aripiprazole, chlorpromazine, clozapine, olanzapine
  - Antiparkinson drugs, such as amantadine, benztropine, trihexyphenidyl
  - Opioids
- Gastrointestinal system:
  - Antidiarrheal drugs, such as atropine, diphenoxylate
  - Antiemetics, such as prochlorperazine, promethazine
  - Antispasmodic drugs, such as belladonna, chlordiazepoxide, hyoscyamine
  - Antivertigo drugs, such as meclizine, scopolamine
  - Antiulcer drugs, such as cimetidine, ranitidine, lansoprazole, omeprazole
- Immune and inflammatory systems:
  - Antihistamines, such as cetirizine, diphenhydramine, loratadine
  - Anti-HIV drugs
  - Anti-infective drugs, such as amphotericin B, ciprofloxacin, clarithromycin, and metronidazole
  - Anti-inflammatory drugs, such as celecoxib, diclofenac, meloxicam
- Musculoskeletal and respiratory systems:
  - Asthma drugs, such as albuterol, ipratropium bromide
  - Muscle relaxants, such as cyclobenzaprine, baclofen, tizanidine
  - Urinary incontinence drugs, such oxybutynin, tolterodine
  - Bisphosphonates, such as alendronate

Although medication-induced hyposalivation is by far the most common cause of dry mouth with eighty percent of the most commonly prescribed medications reportedly causing a decrease in salivary flow, there are two other major causes for decrease in salivation:

- **Radiation-induced hyposalivation** results from radiation therapy used to treat head and neck malignancies. Following several radiation sessions, the salivary glands may become atrophic and possibly non-functional. Usual radiation treatment is 2 GY for 5 consecutive days from 5 up to 8 weeks. A cumulative dose of 60 GY or greater might compromise salivary gland function, requiring lifelong treatment for hyposalivation.

- **Condition-induced hyposalivation** can be the result of Sjögren's Disease, an autoimmune disease in which the body's immune system attacks moisture-producing glands, including salivary, damaging the affected glands partially or completely. Women are at a much higher risk than men. Women, typically in their 40s or 50s, make up 90% of affected individuals. Other causes of disease-induced hyposalivation include AIDS/HIV, Alzheimer's disease, anemia, cystic fibrosis, uncontrolled diabetes, graft-versus-host disease, uncontrolled hypertension, lymphoma, menopause, mumps, Parkinson's disease, pregnancy, rheumatoid arthritis, and stroke as well as other diseases.

3 | Treatment Recommendations for Hyposalivation

The goals of treating xerostomia include identifying the possible cause, relieving discomfort, and preventing oral complications, such as dental caries and periodontal infections. Treatment may include: an assessment of the patient's medical history, a clinical examination of the oral cavity, patient education and lifestyle changes, and, pharmacologic interventions.

Pharmacologic Interventions in collaboration with the patient's physician include drug adaptation, drug adjustment, or drug alteration when appropriate:

- **Drug adaptation**: Switching to a morning treatment regimen, for example, avoids nocturnal dry mouth symptoms in patients who are taking anticholinergic medications.
- **Drug adjustment**: A dose reduction achieved by dividing one large dose into two equal doses or reducing a dose altogether might be beneficial in reducing or even preventing xerostomia.
- **Drug alteration**: In patients with depression, for example, switching the antidepressant regimen (in consultation with the specialist) from a tricyclic antidepressant to a selective serotonin-reuptake inhibitor might solve a dry mouth adverse event.

New treatment interventions include salivary stimulants, including chewing, topical fluoride, and saliva substitutes.

4 | Hypersalivation: Etiology and Treatment

Excess salivation or hypersalivation, although not as prevalent as hyposalivation, poses some logistical problems to the dental team especially when performing composite restoration or when taking dental impressions.

Saliva overproduction or sialorrhea can be either medication-induced or condition-induced.

- Medication-induced sialorrhea can be caused by the use of:
  - Cholinergic agonists for the treatment of Alzheimer's disease or myasthenia gravis
  - Acetylcholinesterase inhibitors found in insecticides
  - Antipsychotics, especially clozapine
  - Yohimbine supplements used by athletes to burn fat and improve performance
  - Nicotine supplements available over-the-counter
- Condition-induced sialorrhea include patients suffering from:
  - Parkinson's disease or patients who have had a recent stroke
  - Neurologically impaired children with mental retardation or cerebral palsy
  - Pregnant women
  - Patients with recurrent aphthous stomatitis or with vitamin B3 deficiency
  - Gastroesophageal reflux disease and oral ulcers
- Pharmacologic interventions consist mainly of:
  - Anticholinergic medications accepted for sialorrhea treatment such glycopyrrolate
  - Anticholinergic medications clinically proven to diminish drooling such as hyoscine patches, sublingual ipratropium spray
  - Botulinum toxin A injected into the parotid and submandibular glands

📖 | Suggested Reading

- Turner MD. Dent Clin North Am 2016;60(2):435-43.
- Villa A, Connell CL, Abati S. Ther Clin Risk Manag 2015;11:45-51.
- Spolarich AE. J Evid Based Dent Pract 2014;14 Suppl:87-94.e1.
- Singh ML, Papas A. Dent Clin North Am 2014;58(4):783-96.
- *ADA.org* Oral Health Topic: Xerostomia (Dry Mouth). *http://www.ADA.org/en/member-center/oral-health-topics/xerostomia.* Accessed August 3, 2018
- Hockstein NG, Samadi DS, Gendron K, Handler SD. Am Fam Physician 2004;69(11):2628-34.
- Plemons JM, Al-Hashimi I, Marek CL. J Am Dent Assoc. 2014 Aug;145(8):867-73.

Drug Monograph

The following tables list some of the medications for hyposalivation and hypersalivation commonly used in dentistry today.

NOTE: The sample prescriptions in this handbook represent a general recommendation. Clinicians are responsible to adjust the prescription dose, frequency and length of treatment based on the procedure performed, the medicine prescribed, and the patient conditions such as age, weight, metabolism, liver and renal function.

For Hyposalivation:

Oral Saliva Substitutes

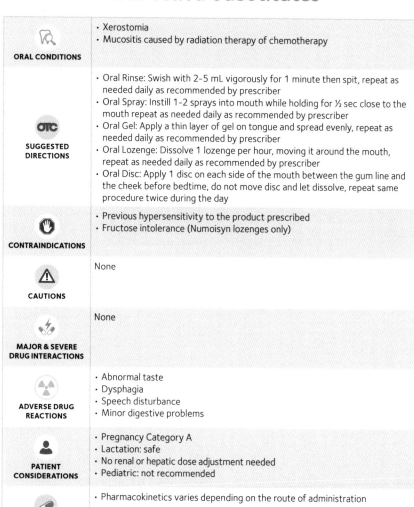

ORAL CONDITIONS	• Xerostomia • Mucositis caused by radiation therapy of chemotherapy
OTC **SUGGESTED DIRECTIONS**	• Oral Rinse: Swish with 2-5 mL vigorously for 1 minute then spit, repeat as needed daily as recommended by prescriber • Oral Spray: Instill 1-2 sprays into mouth while holding for ½ sec close to the mouth repeat as needed daily as recommended by prescriber • Oral Gel: Apply a thin layer of gel on tongue and spread evenly, repeat as needed daily as recommended by prescriber • Oral Lozenge: Dissolve 1 lozenge per hour, moving it around the mouth, repeat as needed daily as recommended by prescriber • Oral Disc: Apply 1 disc on each side of the mouth between the gum line and the cheek before bedtime, do not move disc and let dissolve, repeat same procedure twice during the day
CONTRAINDICATIONS	• Previous hypersensitivity to the product prescribed • Fructose intolerance (Numoisyn lozenges only)
CAUTIONS	None
MAJOR & SEVERE DRUG INTERACTIONS	None
ADVERSE DRUG REACTIONS	• Abnormal taste • Dysphagia • Speech disturbance • Minor digestive problems
PATIENT CONSIDERATIONS	• Pregnancy Category A • Lactation: safe • No renal or hepatic dose adjustment needed • Pediatric: not recommended
DRUG CONSIDERATIONS	• Pharmacokinetics varies depending on the route of administration

Cevimeline
Tablets: 30 mg

ORAL CONDITIONS	• Sjögren Disease
SAMPLE PRESCRIPTION	• Take 1 tablet (30 mg) 3 times per day for at least 6 weeks (126 tablets)
CONTRAINDICATIONS	• Cevimeline hypersensitivity • Asthmatic patients with uncontrolled asthma • Patients with narrow-angle glaucoma • Patients with acute iritis
CAUTIONS	• Patients with significant cardiovascular diseases • Patients with controlled asthma, COPD, chronic bronchitis • Patients with cholelithiasis or biliary tract disease • Patients with a history of nephrolithiasis
MAJOR & SEVERE DRUG INTERACTIONS	This drug ↑ the effects of beta blockers such as atenolol, bisoprolol, metoprolol The following medications ↑ the concentration of the drug • Antibiotics such as erythromycin, clarithromycin • Antifungals such as fluconazole, ketoconazole • Antivirals such as darunavir, ritonavir • Antacids such as cimetidine • Food such as grapefruit The following medications ↓ the concentration of the drug • Anti-inflammatory such as prednisone, dexamethasone • Anticonvulsant such as carbamazepine • Antimigraine such as butalbital • Natural products such as St. John's wort The following medications ↑ the concentration of the drug, however, ↓ the cholinergic effects (less salivation): • Antidepressants such as amitriptyline • General anesthetics such as vecuronium bromide, cisatracurium besilate • Antidiarrheal drugs such as atropine • Antispasmodic drugs such as belladonna • Antihistamines such as diphenhydramine • Urinary incontinence drugs such as oxybutynin, tolterodine • Asthma drugs such as ipratropium • Muscle relaxants such as cyclobenzaprine
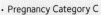 **ADVERSE DRUG REACTIONS**	Common reactions: • Sweating • Headache • Sinusitis, rhinitis • Upper respiratory infection • Nausea Less common reactions: • Delirium, tremor, dizziness • Angina, bronchitis, coughing • Vomiting, dyspepsia, abdominal pain • Asthenia, pain, arthralgia, back pain
PATIENT CONSIDERATIONS	• Pregnancy Category C • Lactation: stop breastfeeding while on medication • Pediatric: not recommended • Elderly: use with caution • No renal or hepatic dose adjustment needed • Don't take with a high fat diet • Drink plenty of water
DRUG CONSIDERATIONS	• Bioavailability: food decreases rate and extent of absorption • Peak serum time: 1.5-2 hr • Protein bound: <20% • Half-life: 5 hr • Excretion: urine 97%, feces 0.5%

Pilocarpine
Tablets: 5 mg, 7.5 mg

ORAL CONDITIONS	• Radiation-induced hyposalivation • Sjögren Disease
SAMPLE PRESCRIPTION	• Take 1 tablet (5 mg) 4 times per day for at least 6 weeks (168 tablets)
CONTRAINDICATIONS	• Pilocarpine hypersensitivity • Asthmatic patients with uncontrolled asthma • Patients with narrow-angle glaucoma • Patients with acute iritis
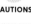**CAUTIONS**	• Patients with significant cardiovascular diseases • Patients with controlled asthma, COPD, chronic bronchitis • Patients with cholelithiasis or biliary tract disease • Patients with a history of nephrolithiasis

MAJOR & SEVERE DRUG INTERACTIONS	• The drug ↑ the effects of beta blockers such as atenolol, bisoprolol, metoprolol
	• The following medications ↑ the concentration of the drug; however, they ↓ the cholinergic effects (less salivation):
	  - Antidepressants, such as amitriptyline
	  - General anesthetics such as vecuronium bromide, cisatracurium besilate
	  - Antidiarrheal drugs such as atropine
	  - Antispasmodic drugs such as belladonna
	  - Antihistamines such as diphenhydramine
	  - Urinary Incontinence drugs such as oxybutynin, tolterodine
	  - Asthma drugs, such as ipratropium bromide
	  - Muscle relaxants, such as cyclobenzaprine

ADVERSE DRUG REACTIONS	Common reactions: • Sweating (29-68%) • Dizziness, flushing, headache • Chills • Rhinitis • Urinary frequency Less common reactions: • Confusion, decreased visual acuity, amblyopia, lacrimation • Bradycardia, hypotension, tachycardia, hypertension • Nausea, vomiting, dyspepsia, diarrhea • Asthenia, pain
PATIENT CONSIDERATIONS	• Pregnancy Category C • Lactation: consider alternative • Pediatric: not recommended • No renal dose adjustment needed, however monitor patients with renal impairment • Hepatic dose adjustment needed in moderately impaired patients reduce frequency to twice a day dosage, and contraindicated in severely impaired patients. • Don't take with a high fat diet • Drink plenty of water
DRUG CONSIDERATIONS	• Bioavailability: high fat meal decreases rate and extent of absorption • Peak serum time: 0.85-1.25 hr • Protein bound: none • Half-life: 0.76-1.35 hr • Excretion: urine

For Hypersalivation:

Glycopyrrolate
Tablets: 1 mg, 1.5 mg, 2 mg · Liquid: 1 mg/5 mL

ORAL CONDITIONS
- Chronic drooling (patients 3-16 years old)

SAMPLE PRESCRIPTION
- Take ½-1 tablet (1 mg-2 mg) 3 times per day for 1 week (11-21 tablets)

CONTRAINDICATIONS
- Glycopyrrolate hypersensitivity
- Patients with narrow-angle glaucoma
- Patients with myasthenia gravis
- Patients with obstructive uropathy

CAUTIONS
- Patients with hyperthyroidism
- Patients with ulcerative colitis or hiatal hernia
- Patients with high fever

MAJOR & SEVERE DRUG INTERACTIONS

The drug ↑ the concentration of the following:
- Potassium salts such as K chloride, K phosphate, and K citrate
- Bronchodilators such as tiotropium, ipratropium
- The hypoglycemia drug glucagon
- Thiazide diuretics such as hydrochlorothiazide (HCTZ), metolazone

ADVERSE DRUG REACTIONS

Common reactions:
- Constipation, urinary retention
- Dry mouth, flushing
- Blurred vision,
- Palpitation, hyperthermia

Less common reactions:
- Tachycardia, cardiac arrhythmia
- Angioedema, paradoxical bronchospasm

PATIENT CONSIDERATIONS
- Pregnancy Category B
- Lactation: use with caution
- Pediatric: FDA approved at 0.1 mg/kg 3 times a day
- No renal or hepatic dose adjustment needed
- Take drug 1 hour before meal or 2 hours after meal

DRUG CONSIDERATIONS
- Peak serum time: 30-45 min
- Half-life: 3 hr
- Excretion: urine (85%), bile (<5%)

Other Treatments for Hypersalivation:

RX MEDICATION	SAMPLE PRESCRIPTION	PATIENT CONSIDERATIONS	ADVERSE DRUG REACTIONS
Hyoscine hydrobromide patch (Scopolamine (Transderm-Scop 1.5 mg)	Apply 1 patch (1.5 mg) every 3 days	Be cautious with: · Glaucoma patients · Patients with urinary retention · Elderly patients with kidney problems · Pregnant women	· Pruritus at patch site · urinary retention · irritability · blurred vision · dizziness · glaucoma
Atropine 1% ophthalmic solution for sublingual use	Instill 2 to 4 drops sublingually every 2 to 4 hours a day as needed (15 mL bottle)	Sublingual use of an ophthalmic solution	· Constipation · xerostomia · blurred vision · urinary retention
Ipratropium bromide 0.03% nasal spray for sublingual use	Squirt 2 to 4 sprays sublingually every 6 hours a day as needed (30 mL bottle)	Sublingual use of a nasal solution	· Xerostomia · blurred vision · taste perversion
Propantheline 15 mg	Take 1 tablet (15 mg) every 8 hours a day as needed	Take tablet 30 min before meals or 2 hours after meals	· Constipation · xerostomia · blurred vision · urinary retention · hyperactivity
Botulinum toxin A 100 U per vial	Inject 10 to 40 units into each submandibular and parotid gland	Use when other alternatives fail	· Pain at injection site · high xerostomia

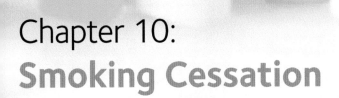

Chapter 10:
Smoking Cessation

Kathleen Ziegler, PharmD

Overview

All forms of tobacco used in the United States have oral health consequences, placing the dentist in a unique position to offer discussion about tobacco use recognition, prevention, and cessation. Cigarette smoking can lead to a variety of adverse oral effects, including gingival recession, impaired healing following periodontal therapy, oral cancer, mucosal lesions (e.g., oral leukoplakia, nicotine stomatitis), periodontal disease, and tooth staining. Use of smokeless tobacco is associated with increased risks of oral cancer and oral mucosal lesions (e.g., oral leukoplakia). Smokeless tobacco use also causes oral conditions such as gingival keratosis, tooth discoloration, halitosis, enamel erosion, gingival recession, alveolar bone damage, periodontal disease, tooth loss, and coronal or root-surface dental caries due to sugars added to the product. Second-hand smoke has been linked to periodontal disease.

1 │ Learn the 5 As

Because of the oral health implications of tobacco use, dental practices may provide a uniquely effective setting for tobacco use recognition, prevention, and cessation. Health-care professionals, including dental professionals, can help smokers quit by consistently identifying patients who smoke, advising them to quit, and offering them information about cessation treatment. The U.S. Department of Health and Human Services Agency for Healthcare Research and Quality has published a five-step algorithm for health-care professionals to use when engaging patients who are dependent on nicotine called "The 5As" (Five Major Steps to Intervention. *http://www.ahrq.gov/ professionals/clinicians-providers/guidelines-recommendations/tobacco/5steps.html*).

The five steps are:

1. **Ask**: Identify and document tobacco use status for every patient at every visit.

2. **Advise**: In a clear, strong, and personalized manner, urge every tobacco user to quit.

3. **Assess**: Is the tobacco user willing to make a quit attempt at this time?

4. **Assist**: For the patient willing to make a quit attempt, use counseling and pharmacotherapy to help him or her quit.

5. **Arrange**: Schedule follow-up contact, in person or by telephone, preferably within the first week after the quit date.

The 2008 U.S. Public Health Service clinical practice guideline for treating tobacco use and dependence found that counseling or medication are effective when used by themselves for treating tobacco dependence; however, the combination of counseling plus medication was more effective than either method alone.

In the United States, telephone counseling is available free through a system of state-based quit lines accessible with one toll-free number (1-800-QUIT-NOW [784-8669]).

2 | Pharmacologic Interventions

According to the Centers for Disease Control and Prevention, use of cessation medications is appropriate for most adult smokers, with the exception of:

- pregnant women
- light smokers (i.e., persons who smoke fewer than 5 to 10 cigarettes daily)
- persons with specific medical contraindications (e.g., seizure disorders)

Nicotine-replacement therapy, bupropion (an atypical antidepressant), and varenicline (a selective nicotine receptor partial agonist) are first-line pharmacologic therapies recommended by the U.S. Department of Health and Human Services to assist with smoking cessation.

A 2014 summary of 12 Cochrane reviews looking at efficacy and harms of pharmacologic therapies for smoking cessation used network meta-analysis to make direct and indirect comparisons of efficacy between nicotine-replacement therapy, bupropion, and varenicline for smoking cessation. The review found higher abstinence rates with nicotine-replacement therapies (17.6%) and bupropion (19.1%), compared with placebo (10.6%). Varenicline (27.6%) or a combination of nicotine-replacement therapies (e.g., longer-acting patch plus short-acting inhaler, 31.5%) were the most effective approaches for achieving smoking cessation. The analysis found that none of the therapies was associated with an increased rate of serious adverse events.

📖 | **Suggested Reading**

- Cahill K, Stevens S, Lancaster T. Pharmacological treatments for smoking cessation. JAMA 2014;311(2):193-4.
- Couch ET, Chaffee BW, Gansky SA, Walsh MM. The changing tobacco landscape: What dental professionals need to know. J Am Dent Assoc 2016;147(7):561-9.
- Drugs for tobacco dependence. Med Lett Drugs Ther 2016;58(1489):27-31
- Jamal A, King BA, Neff LJ, et al. Current Cigarette Smoking Among Adults - United States, 2005-2015. MMWR Morb Mortal Wkly Rep 2016;65(44):1205-11.
- Levy JM, Abramowicz S. Medications to Assist in Tobacco Cessation for Dental Patients. Dent Clin North Am 2016;60(2):533-40.
- National Institute on Drug Abuse. Research Report Series: Tobacco/Nicotine (NIH Publication Number 16-4342). National Institutes of Health.

Drug Monograph

The following tables list prescription and non-prescription medications commonly used in dentistry today to assist patients with tobacco cessation.

NOTE: The sample prescriptions in this handbook represent a general recommendation. Clinicians are responsible to adjust the prescription dose, frequency and length of treatment based on the procedure performed, the medicine prescribed, and the patient conditions such as age, weight, metabolism, liver and renal function.

Nicotine Replacement Therapies
Intranasal: 0.5 mg · Inhaled: 10 mg · Gum/Lozenges: 2 mg, 4 mg
Transdermal: 5 mg, 7 mg, 10 mg, 14 mg, 15 mg, 21 mg

ORAL CONDITIONS	· Smoking cessation
SAMPLE PRESCRIPTION	· Intranasal Nicotine: Squirt 1 to 2 sprays (1x 0.5 mg to 2x 0.5 mg) per nostril every hour, up to a maximum of 80 sprays per day *Maximum daily dosage of 40 mg or 1/2 bottle per day* *Maximum duration of therapy 3 months* · Inhaled Nicotine: Inhale the content of 6 to 12 cartridges (6x 10 mg to 12x 10 mg) per day as needed up to a maximum of 16 cartridges per day *Each cartridge has 10 mg of nicotine but only 4 mg are delivered* *Recommended duration between 6 to12 weeks*

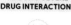 **SUGGESTED DIRECTIONS**	· **Transdermal Nicotine:**
	For patients smoking more than 10 cigarettes/day
	  – One 21-mg patch/day x 6 weeks, then
	  – One 14-mg patch/day x 2 weeks, then
	  – One 7-mg patch/day x 2 weeks
	For patients smoking less than 10 cigarettes/day (or weight <45 kg)
	  – One 14-mg patch/day x 6 weeks, then
	  – One 7-mg patch/day x 2 weeks
	· **Nicotine Gums and Lozenges:**
	For patients who smoke within 30 minutes of waking up
	  – One 4-mg piece every 1 to 2 hours x 6 weeks, then
	  – One 4-mg piece every 2 to 4 hours x 3 weeks, then
	  – One 4-mg piece every 4 to 8 hours x 3 weeks
	For patients who smoke 30 minutes after waking up
	  – One 2-mg piece every 1 to 2 hours x 6 weeks, then
	  – One 2-mg piece every 2 to 4 hours x 3 weeks, then
	  – One 2-mg piece every 4 to 8 hours x 3 weeks

CONTRAINDICATIONS	· Hypersensitivity to nicotine or to any component of the product
CAUTIONS	· Patients with cardiovascular or peripheral vascular diseases, including coronary heart disease, serious cardiac arrhythmias, or vasospastic diseases · Patients with peptic ulcer disease
MAJOR & SEVERE DRUG INTERACTIONS	· Effect of smoking cessation on other drugs: Pharmacokinetics or pharmacodynamics of certain drugs (e.g., theophylline, warfarin, and insulin) may be altered, necessitating dose adjustment.
ADVERSE DRUG REACTIONS	Common reactions: · Headache · Nausea, vomiting, diarrhea · Abdominal pain · Oral mucosal, oropharyngeal, nasal, or skin irritation Less common reactions: · Vivid dreams, insomnia
PATIENT CONSIDERATIONS	· Pregnancy Category D · Lactation: weigh the risk of exposure to nicotine from either nicotine replacement therapy or nicotine from continued smoking by the mother and contamination of breast milk with other components of tobacco smoke · Pediatric: not evaluated · Keep out of reach of children and pets · Do not smoke while on nicotine replacement therapy as nicotine overdose can occur · Intranasal use not recommended in patients with chronic nasal disorders (e.g., allergy, rhinitis, nasal polyps, and sinusitis) · Patients with preexisting asthma may develop bronchospasm
DRUG CONSIDERATIONS	· Pharmacokinetics varies depending on the route of administration

Bupropion HCl SR (Zyban®)

Tablets: 150 mg

ORAL CONDITIONS	• Smoking cessation
SAMPLE PRESCRIPTION	• Take 1 tablet (150 mg) daily for 3 days then take 1 tablet (150 mg) twice a day thereafter for at least 12 weeks (165 tablets)

BLACK BOX WARNING: Increased risk of suicidal thinking and behavior in children, adolescents, and young adults taking antidepressants; monitor for worsening and emergence of suicidal thoughts and behaviors.

CONTRAINDICATIONS	• Hypersensitivity to bupropion • Seizure disorder • Current or prior diagnosis of bulimia or anorexia nervosa • Patients abruptly discontinuing alcohol, benzodiazepines, barbiturates, or antiepileptic drugs • Patients receiving monoamine oxidase inhibitors, linezolid, or IV methylene blue
CAUTIONS	• Patients with bipolar disorder: monitor for these symptoms • Psychotic patients with previous neuropsychiatric reactions • Patients with angle-closure glaucoma

MAJOR & SEVERE DRUG INTERACTIONS	• This drug increases the concentration of the following drugs:
	  - antidepressants (e.g., venlafaxine, fluoxetine, sertraline),
	  - antipsychotics (e.g., haloperidol, risperidone,),
	  - beta-blockers (e.g., metoprolol),
	  - Type 1C antiarrhythmics (e.g., propafenone, flecainide).
	• The following medications decrease the concentration of the drug:
	  - ritonavir, lopinavir, efavirenz,
	  - carbamazepine, phenobarbital or phenytoin; (dose increase may be necessary based on clinical response but should not exceed the maximum recommended dose)
	• Bupropion may decrease plasma digoxin levels; monitor digoxin levels.
	• Dopaminergic drugs (e.g., levodopa and amantadine): CNS toxicity can occur when used concomitantly with bupropion.
	• Monoamine oxidase inhibitors: Increased risk of hypertensive reactions can occur when used concomitantly

ADVERSE DRUG REACTIONS	Common reactions: • Insomnia • Rhinitis • Dry mouth • Dizziness • Nervous disturbance or anxiety • Nausea, constipation • Arthralgia Less common reactions: • Psychosis, neuropsychiatric reactions • Hypertension • Seizure
PATIENT CONSIDERATIONS	• Pregnancy Category C • Lactation: exercise caution as the drug is excreted in human milk • Pediatric: use not established • Consider a reduced dose and/or dosing frequency in patients with renal impairment • In patients with moderate to severe hepatic impairment, the maximum dose is 150 mg every other day. In patients with mild hepatic impairment, consider reducing the dose and/or frequency of dosing. • Limit or avoid using alcohol during treatment • May be taken with or without food • Do not crush, divide, or chew the tablet, as this may lead to an increased risk of adverse effect, including seizures
DRUG CONSIDERATIONS	• Peak serum time: 3 hr • Half-life: 21 (+/-9) hr • Excretion: 87% urine, 10% feces; only 0.5% of the oral dose was excreted as unchanged bupropion

Varenicline Tartrate (Chantix®)

Tablets: 0.5 mg, 1 mg

ORAL CONDITIONS	• Smoking cessation
SAMPLE PRESCRIPTION	• Varenicline starting pack: Take 1 tablet (0.5 mg) daily for 3 days then take 1 tablet (0.5 mg) twice a day for another 4 days (11 tablets) • Varenicline continuation pack: Take 1 tablet (1 mg) twice a day for 12 weeks (168 tablets) **NOTE**: Patient may quit smoking between days 8 and 35 of treatment. An additional 12 weeks of treatment is recommended for those who successfully quit to increase likelihood of long-term abstinence
CONTRAINDICATIONS	• History of hypersensitivity or skin reactions to varenicline
CAUTIONS	• Patients with a history of seizures or neuropsychiatric problems
MAJOR & SEVERE DRUG INTERACTIONS	• No meaningful drug interactions
ADVERSE DRUG REACTIONS	Common reactions: • Nausea • Abnormal (e.g., vivid, unusual, or strange) dreams • Constipation • Flatulence • Vomiting Less common reactions: • Neuropsychiatric adverse events • Cardiovascular events • Seizure
PATIENT CONSIDERATIONS	• Pregnancy Category C: available human data in pregnant women are not sufficient to inform a drug-associated risk • Lactation: unknown if present in human milk, discontinue drug while breastfeeding • Pediatric: use not established • Dosage adjustment required in patients with severe renal impairment • Limit or avoid using alcohol during treatment
DRUG CONSIDERATIONS	• Oral bioavailability is unaffected by food or time-of-day dosing. • Peak serum time: 3-4 hr • Low plasma protein binding (<20%) • Half-life: ~24 hr • Excretion: 92% unchanged in urine

Chapter 11:
Supplemental Drugs: Allergy Management, Herbals in Dental Health, Skeletal Muscle Relaxants

Lakshmanan Suresh, DDS, MS, PhD, D(ABMLI), D(ABOMP) and Lida Radfar, DDS, MS

Overview

1 | Allergy Management

Ascertaining the nature of the allergic reaction as being minor (non-life threatening) versus major (life threatening) is the first step in allergy management. If the reactions are limited to the skin, such as rashes and hives, then it is considered minor and non-life threatening. If the symptoms involve the life threatening symptoms such as swelling of the tongue, wheezing and difficulty breathing, it is considered major allergic reaction.

Minor skin reactions are managed by administrations of antihistamine such as diphenhydramine (Benadryl) 25-50 mg (dosage depends on age) and by intramuscular (IM) injection of diphenhydramine in the deltoid muscle using a 50 mg/mL concentration (0.5-1.0 mL) in more severe reactions. As the histamines circulate in the blood for three days after the initial attack, the patients also should be taking oral diphenhydramine 25-50 mg (dosage depends on the age but usually 25 mg for children and 50 mg for adults) four times daily for 3 days, in addition to the diphenhydramine IM injection administered during the initial allergy attack.

Major allergy attacks are usually life threatening and require the **A**irway, **B**reathing, **C**irculation, **D**isability, **E**xposure (ABCDE) approach described in the flowchart. A major allergy attack usually is an anaphylactic attack and typically, there is a rapid onset of signs and symptoms following allergen exposure. Early signs and symptoms include (For more on this topic, refer to Section 3: Emergency Drug Management.)

📖 | Suggested Reading

- Becker DE. Drug allergies and implications for dental practice. Anesth Prog 2013;60(4):188-97.
- Nanavati RS, Kumar M, Modi TG, Kale H. Anaphylactic shock management in dental clinics: An overview. J Int Clin Dent Res Organ 2013;5(1):36-9.
- Panel NS. Guidelines for the diagnosis and management of food allergy in the United States: report of the NIAID-sponsored expert panel. J Allergy Clin Immunol 2010;126(6):S1-58. (*https://www.ncbi.nlm.nih.gov/pmc/articles/PMC4241964*)

Table 1. Acute Allergy Management

Perform Primary Assessment	• Remove allergen
	• Perform ABCDE assessment
	  – **A**irway: swelling, airway stridor, check for obstruction
	  – **B**reathing: rapid respiratory rate, cyanosis
	  – **C**irculation: low blood pressure, pallor
	  – **D**isability: reduced consciousness, dilated pupils, drowsiness
	  – **E**xposure: adequate skin exposure for examination
	• Call 911

Diagnosis	**Major – Life Threatening** • airway compromised • wheezing • swelling of tongue or throat
Treatment	
Epinephrine (IM)	• Infants/Children <15 kg: exact weight based dose or 0.15 mg if patient rapidly deteriorating • Children 15-29 kg: 0.15 mg (0.15 mL of 1 mg/mL solution) • Patients 30-50 kg: 0.3 mg (0.3 mL of 1 mg/mL solution) • Patients >50 kg: 0.5 mg (0.5 mL of 1 mg/mL solution) *(repeat after 5-15 minutes if no response)*
IV Fluids	• Adults: 500-1,000 mL • Children: crystalloid 20 mL/kg
Diphenhydramine	• Adults: 25-50 mg intravenously over 5 minutes, may be repeated up to a maximum dose of 400 mg per 24 hrs • Children <50 kg: 1 mg/kg (maximum 50 mg) intravenously over 5 minutes, may be repeated up to a maximum dose of 200 mg per 24 hrs

Albuterol	• Via metered inhaler:
	  – Adults: 8 puffs
	  – Children: 4-8 puffs
	• Via nebulized solution:
	  – Adults: 3 mL
	  – Children: 1.5 mL
	(administer over 20 minutes or continuously as needed)

2 | Herbals in Dental Health

Herbals are medicinal products derived from plants. Homeopathy uses products that are of plant, animal and chemical origin in small doses to treat or prevent diseases progression. Since dentists may encounter patients who use herbals, it is important to understand the interactions of commonly used herbal supplements. The table below lists and summarizes most common herbals products and their interactions with other medications used in dentistry. Only selected and commonly used herbal medications and their adverse effects in dental uses are discussed.

HERBAL SUPPLEMENT	INDICATIONS	ADVERSE DRUG REACTIONS	DRUG INTERACTIONS
Table 2. Common Herbal Supplements			
Aloe	• Burns • Skin/mucosal irritation		• May potentiate anticoagulant therapy by reducing absorption of vitamin K from the gut
Dong quai	• Pain management • Gynecological conditions		• May interfere with blood clotting and can potentiate antithrombotic effects of warfarin/aspirin/clopidogrel
Echinacea	• Infection • Boost immune system	• Tongue numbness • Aggravation of autoimmune progressive conditions such as lupus and multiple sclerosis	
Ephedra	• Respiratory conditions • Weight loss	• Hypertension • Anxiety • Dysrhythmias	
Feverfew	• Toothaches • Fever • Migraines • Arthritis • Gynecological conditions	• Mouth ulcers • Dry mouth • Altered taste	• May interfere with blood clotting and can potentiate antithrombotic effects of warfarin/aspirin/clopidogrel
Fish oils	• Cardiac health • Skin disorders • Diabetes • Headache • Ulcerative colitis		• May interfere with blood clotting and can potentiate antithrombotic effects of warfarin/aspirin/clopidogrel
Garlic	• Antimicrobial • Anti-asthmatic • Anti-inflammatory • Anti-lipidemic • Lower blood pressure		• May interfere with blood clotting and can potentiate antithrombotic effects of warfarin/aspirin/clopidogrel

Table 2. Common Herbal Supplements			
HERBAL SUPPLEMENT	**INDICATIONS**	**ADVERSE DRUG REACTIONS**	**DRUG INTERACTIONS**
Ginger	• Antioxidant • Arthritis • Antimicrobial for digestive disorders • Indigestion		• May interfere with blood clotting and can potentiate antithrombotic effects of warfarin/aspirin/clopidogrel
Gingko	• Epilepsy • Nerve damage		• May interfere with blood clotting and can potentiate antithrombotic effects of warfarin/aspirin/clopidogrel
Ginseng	• Increased circulation • Cardiovascular disease		• May interfere with blood clotting and can potentiate antithrombotic effects of warfarin/aspirin/clopidogrel/NSAIDs
Goldenseal	• Digestive disorders • Wound healing	• Increases saliva • Can cause increase in blood pressure at high doses	
Grapeseed extract	• Increased circulation • Skin health		
Red pepper	• Increased circulation • Treatment of burning tongue		
St. John's wort	• Depression • Analgesic • Anti-inflammatory	• Increased photosensitivity • Inhibits MAO inhibitors	• May interfere with blood clotting and can potentiate antithrombotic effects of warfarin/aspirin/clopidogrel
Vitamin A	• Acne	• Excessive intake can cause hepatotoxicity, delayed wound healing and birth defects	
Vitamin D	• Osteoporosis	• Excessive intake can cause calcifications and enamel hypoplasia	
Vitamin E	• Antioxidant		• May interfere with blood clotting and can potentiate antithrombotic effects of warfarin/aspirin/clopidogrel

📖 | **Suggested Reading**

- Abebe W. An overview of herbal supplement utilization with particular emphasis on possible interactions with dental drugs and oral manifestations. J Dent Hyg 2002;77(1):37-46.
- Cohan RP, Jacobsen PL. Herbal supplements: considerations in dental practice. J Calif Dent Assoc 2000;28(8):600-10.
- Little JW. Complementary and alternative medicine: impact on dentistry. Oral Surg Oral Med Oral Pathol Oral Radiol Endod 2004;98(2):137-45.
- Wu CH, Wang CC, Kennedy J. Changes in herb and dietary supplement use in the U.S. adult population: a comparison of the 2002 and 2007 National Health Interview Surveys. Clin Ther 2011;33(11):1749-58.

3 | Skeletal Muscle Relaxants

Skeletal muscle relaxants can be classified based on the mechanism of action and indication of use as antispasticity and antispasmodic agents. There are a few drugs that can act as both antispastic and antispasmodic agents. The primary use of skeletal muscle relaxants in the dental office is to relieve anxiety, post procedural trismus, and muscle spasms of the head and neck including temporomandibular disorders. These agents often are used in conjunction with heat, physical therapy, rest, and analgesics. Some of these agents have anxiolytic properties that may help reduce muscle tension.

- **Antispasticity agents** act directly on skeletal muscles to improve muscle tone (reduce stiffness and uncontrolled movements). The antispasticity medications are mainly used in neurological conditions such as cerebral palsy, multiple sclerosis, and spinal cord injuries. Baclofen and dantrolene are the two main medications that belong to this class of drugs.

- **Antispasmodic agents** act on the neuromuscular junctions or directly on the brain stem to decrease muscle spasms. The main drugs are benzodiazepines, carisoprodol, cyclobenzaprine, metaxalone, and methocarbamol. Benzodiazepines are used as sedatives, anxiolytics, and anticonvulsants, while the antispasmodics are commonly prescribed for the reduction of muscle spasms.

- **Antispastic and antispasmodic agents** alleviate both spasms and spasticity. Tizanidine, is a drug can that act as both an antispastic and antispasmodic agent.

See Table 3 on page 100 for more information about skeletal muscle relaxants.

📖 | **Suggested Reading**

- Beebe FA, Barkin RL, Barkin S. A clinical and pharmacologic review of skeletal muscle relaxants for musculoskeletal conditions. Am J Ther 2005;12:151-71.
- Clark G, Sahai-Srivaastava S. Skeletal muscle relaxants and antispasticity drugs for orofacial pain disorders. Orofacial Pain: a guide to medications and management. Oxford: Wiley-Blackwell. 2012 Mar 20:115-28.
- Witenko C, Moorman-Li R, Motycka C, et al. Considerations for the appropriate use of skeletal muscle relaxants for the management of acute low back pain. PT 2014;39(6):427.

Table 3. Skeletal Muscle Relaxants

RX MEDICATION	SAMPLE PRESCRIPTION*	ADVERSE DRUG REACTIONS	CAUTIONS
Antispasticity Agents			
Baclofen 5 mg	Take 1 to 2 tablets 3 times a day for 5 days as needed (15-30 tablets) *May increase by 5 mg every 3 days, but do not exceed 20 mg, 4 times/day (80 mg daily)*	• Drowsiness • Dizziness • Nausea • Weakness/fatigue • Confusion • Hypotension • Increased urinary frequency • Xerostomia	**BLACK BOX WARNING:** For long term therapy: Do not stop drug abruptly, titrate down over several weeks
Antispasmodic Agents			
Carisoprodol 250 or 350 mg	Take 1 tablet 4 times a day for 5 days as needed (20 tablets)	• Drowsiness • Dizziness • Headache	• Do not use longer than 3 weeks • Avoid alcohol while on medication
Cyclobenzaprine 5 mg	Take 1 to 2 tablets 3 times a day for 5 days as needed (15-30 tablets)	• Drowsiness • Xerostomia • Dizziness • Blurred vision	• Do not use longer than 3 weeks • Do not use comcommitantly with MAOIs such as selegiline, rosagiline
Metaxaolone 800 mg	Take 1 tablet 3-4 times a day for 5 days as needed (15-20 tablets)	• Drowsiness • Dizziness • Skin rash • Nausea/vomiting • Hemolytic anemia • Jaundice	• Contraindicated in patients with renal or hepatic impairement
Orphenadrine 100 mg	Take 1 tablet 2 times a day for 3-5 days as needed (6-10 tablets)	• Drowsiness • Xerostomia • Dizziness • Tachycardia • Blurred vision • Urinary retention	• Derivative of diphenydramine • Intended for short-term use
Antispasicity and Antispasmodic Agents			
Tizanidine 2 mg	Take 1 to 2 tablets 3 times a day for 5 days as needed (15-30 tablets) *May titrate to optimal effect, but do not exceed 36 mg/day Single doses >16 mg have not been studied*	• Drowsiness • Xerostomia • Dizziness • Hypotension • Hepatic injury • Bradycardia • Weakness • Hallucinations	• Oral contraceptives reduce tizanidine clearance by 50%

* The sample prescriptions in this handbook represent a general recommendation. Clinicians are responsible to adjust the prescription dose, frequency and length of treatment based on the procedure performed, the medicine prescribed, and the patient conditions such as age, weight, metabolism, liver and renal function.

Chapter 12:
OTC Products with the ADA Seal of Acceptance

Louis Erazo, BS

Overview

The American Dental Association (ADA) Seal of Acceptance Program is the gold standard for the safety and efficacy of over-the-counter (OTC) dental products for the advancement of oral health. Manufacturers commit significant resources to clinical trials and laboratory testing to demonstrate that the product is safe, as well as effective in its therapeutic claims. It is important for your patients to know that when they see the ADA Seal on a product, that product has been objectively evaluated by an independent body of scientific experts, the ADA Council on Scientific Affairs.

The following sections will focus on oral health care topics that have OTC options available within the ADA Seal of Acceptance Program. Making your patients aware of these options will allow them to be more informed consumers and aid them in choosing the best products to incorporate into their daily oral hygiene regimen. More information about the ADA Seal of Acceptance Program can be found at *www.ada.org/seal*.

1 | Dental Caries

One of the best preventive measure against caries is daily fluoride use. The ADA recommends brushing with an ADA Accepted toothpaste containing fluoride twice a day as well as cleaning between the teeth once a day to prevent cavities. In addition, the regular use of a fluoride-containing mouth rinse in your patient's daily oral hygiene regimen can provide added protection against caries. All ADA Accepted mouth rinses intended to prevent cavities meet U.S. and international safety standards, including pH. A final recommendation to your patients in helping to reduce their caries risk is to maintain a diet low in added sugars.

Tables 1a and b list OTC products with the ADA Seal of Acceptance (current as of publication date, 2018) for the prevention of caries. Including any of these dentifrices in their daily oral health care routine can help patients maximize efforts in cavity protection and prevention. Patients who are at increased risk for caries or gingivitis might consider adding an ADA Accepted mouthrinse.

2 | Plaque and Gingivitis

Early intervention is advised to stop the progression of gingivitis into periodontitis. If the patient's condition is at an early stage, there are ADA Seal products — specifically toothpastes and mouthrinses — you can recommend to help prevent progression of the disease. All ADA Accepted antiseptic mouth rinses meet U.S. and international safety standards, including pH.

Tables 2a and b and Tables 6a-d list OTC products with the ADA Seal of Acceptance (current as of publication date, 2018) used to treat and prevent plaque and gingivitis. Including any of these products in their daily oral health care routine can help patients increase protection from and prevention of plaque and gingivitis.

3 | Dentinal Hypersensitivity

There are a variety of treatment options available for patients affected by sensitive teeth. The appropriate course of action often depends on the severity of your patient's hypersensitivity and whether or not there are other contributing factors to their condition e.g.gastroesophageal reflux disease, recent dental bleaching, aggressive oral hygiene practices, etc.). All ADA Accepted mouth rinses intended to manage hypersensitivity meet U.S. and international safety standards, including pH.

Table 3 lists OTC toothpastes with the ADA Seal of Acceptance (current as of publication date, 2018) for helping to manage dentinal hypersensitivity. Including any of these products in their daily oral health care routine can help patients with their sensitive teeth.

4 | Erosion

The main cause of erosion is the sustained contact of tooth enamel to an acidic environment. This can be introduced into the oral cavity by frequent consumption of acidic foods and beverages as well as other health factors such as gastroesophageal reflux disease or GERD.

The demineralization of tooth enamel can occur when the pH inside the oral environment is below 5.5. Erosion will begin as tooth surface softening that could eventually lead to the irreversible loss of tooth enamel. Once tooth enamel is lost, it cannot be regenerated and can lead to a host of other oral conditions such as tooth decay, cavities, hypersensitivity and tooth loss. Since erosion is a condition that exists in a continuum of stages, there are more treatment options available at the early stages than when the disease has progressed to a point of non-repair.

Early intervention is important in helping prevent or manage erosion in your patients. Patients should understand that reducing the amount of acidic beverages consumed on a daily basis and limiting contact time with these acid challenges is a very effective preventive measure against erosion. All ADA Accepted toothpastes and mouthrinses meet U.S. and international safety standards for pH.

Table 4 lists OTC products with the ADA Seal of Acceptance (current as of publication date, 2018) for dental erosion prevention/management. Including any of these products in their oral health care routine can help patients prevent or manage dental erosion.

5 | Topical Oral Pain Relief Products

Oral pain in the mouth and gums can be a common occurrence for orthodontic patients as well as the general public. Topically applied liquids or gels containing active ingredients intended for the temporarily relief of oral pain is a treatment option for patients experiencing this pain due to mouth sores.

Table 5 lists OTC products with the ADA Seal of Acceptance (current as of publication date, 2018) for topical oral pain relief. Including any of these products in their oral health care routine can help patients temporarily relieve oral pain due to mouth sores.

List of ADA Seal Accepted Products

Below is a list of products with the ADA Seal of Acceptance as of date of this publication (2018) such as OTC dentifrices, mouthrinses and oral pain remedies. Including any of these products in their daily oral health routine can help patients when addressing concerns like caries, plaque and gingivitis, hypersensitivity, erosion or oral pain.

For the most recent listing of ADA Seal Accepted products, refer to the ADA website at ADA.org/seal.

Table 1a. Caries Prevention: Dentifrices	
ADA SEAL ACCEPTED DENTIFRICES	ACTIVE INGREDIENTS
Aim Cavity Protection	Sodium fluoride (0.24%)
AloeSense Toothpaste	Sodium fluoride (0.24%)
Aquafresh for Kids Toothpaste	Sodium monofluorophosphate (0.76%)
Arm & Hammer Dental Care Advance Cleaning Mint Toothpaste with Baking Soda	Sodium fluoride (0.24%)
Benco Dental PRO-SYS Kids Fluoride Toothgel (Bubblegum flavor)	Sodium fluoride (0.24%
Benco Dental PRO-SYS Fluoride Toothgel (Mint flavor)	Sodium fluoride (0.24%)
Cardinal Health Anticavity Toothpaste with Fluoride	Sodium fluoride (0.24%)
CloSYS Sulfate-free Toothpaste	Sodium fluoride (0.24%)
Colgate Cavity Protection Gel	Sodium fluoride (0.24%)
Colgate Cavity Protection Great Regular Flavor Fluoride Toothpaste	Sodium monofluorophosphate (0.76%)
Colgate for Kids Toothpaste	Sodium fluoride (0.24%)
Colgate for Kids Maximum Cavity Protection Toothpaste	Sodium fluoride (0.24%)
Colgate Total Advanced Deep Clean Toothpaste	Sodium fluoride (0.24%)
Colgate Total Advanced Fresh & Whitening Gel	Sodium fluoride (0.24%)
Colgate Total Clean Mint Toothpaste	Sodium fluoride (0.24%)
Colgate Total Mint Stripe Toothpaste	Sodium fluoride (0.24%)
Colgate Total Whitening Gel	Sodium fluoride (0.24%)
Colgate Total Whitening Paste	Sodium fluoride (0.24%)

Table 1a. Caries Prevention: Dentifrices

ADA SEAL ACCEPTED DENTIFRICES	ACTIVE INGREDIENTS
Cool Wave Fresh Mint Gel Fluoride Anticavity Toothpaste	Sodium fluoride (0.24%)
Crest Cavity Protection Toothpaste	Sodium fluoride (0.24%)
Crest Cavity Protection Cool Mint Gel	Sodium fluoride (0.24%)
Crest Kids Sparkle Fun Cavity Protection Toothpaste	Sodium fluoride (0.24%)
Crest Pro-Health Advanced Deep Clean Mint Toothpaste	Stannous fluoride (0.454%)
Crest Pro-Health Extra Whitening Power Toothpaste	Stannous fluoride (0.454%)
Crest Pro-Health Toothpaste (Cool Spearmint, Intense Peppermint flavors)	Stannous fluoride (0.454%)
Crest Tartar Protection Fresh Mint Gel	Sodium fluoride (0.24%)
Crest Tartar Protection Regular Paste	Sodium fluoride (0.24%)
DTI Toothgel (Bubblegum, Bubblegum Saccharin Free, Mint flavors)	Sodium fluoride (0.24%)
DTI Toothpaste (Bubblegum, Mint flavors)	Sodium fluoride (0.24%)
Freshmint Premium Anticavity Toothpaste	Sodium fluoride (0.24%)
Freshmint Premium Anticavity Gel	Sodium fluoride (0.24%)
Hello Kid's Fluoride Toothpaste (Blue Raspberry, Bubblegum flavors)	Sodium fluoride (0.24%)
Hello Mojito Mint Whitening Fluoride Toothpaste	Sodium fluoride (0.24%)
Oraline Fluoride Mint Toothpaste	Sodium fluoride (0.24%)
Oraline Kids Bubblegum Flavored Fluoride Toothpaste	Sodium fluoride (0.24%)
Oraline Kids Bubblegum Flavored Fluoride Toothgel	Sodium fluoride (0.24%)
Oraline Secure Clear Fluoride Mint Toothpaste	Sodium fluoride (0.24%)
Sensodyne Toothpaste (Fresh Impact, Fresh Mint flavors)	Sodium fluoride (0.24%)
Sheffield Fluoride Toothpaste NS# 3415 (Original, Bubblegum, Mint flavors)	Sodium fluoride (0.24%)
Smile Central Dental Bubblegum Fluoride Toothgel	Sodium fluoride (0.24%)
Superba! Fluoride Toothpaste	Sodium fluoride (0.24%)
Tom's of Maine Children's Gel Fruitilicious	Sodium fluoride (0.24%)
Tom's of Maine Natural Baking Soda Fluoride Toothpaste (Peppermint flavor)	Sodium monofluorophosphate (0.76%)
Tom's of Maine Natural Fluoride Toothpaste for Children (Silly Strawberry, Outrageous Orange Mango flavors)	Sodium monofluorophosphate (0.76%)
Tom's of Maine Natural Wicked Cool!	Sodium monofluorophosphate (0.76%)
Tom's of Maine Simply White Clean Mint	Sodium monofluorophosphate (0.76%)
Tom's of Maine Simply White Sweet Mint Gel	Sodium monofluorophosphate (0.76%)
Tom's of Maine Natural Anticavity Fluoride Toothpaste (Spearmint flavor)	Sodium monofluorophosphate (0.76%)

Table 1b. Caries Prevention: Mouthrinses

ADA SEAL ACCEPTED MOUTHRINSES	ACTIVE INGREDIENTS
ACT Anticavity Fluoride Rinse (Cinnamon, Mint flavors)	Sodium fluoride (0.05%)
ACT Kid's Anticavity Fluoride Rinse (Bubblegum, SpongeBob Ocean Berry flavors)	Sodium fluoride (0.05%)
ACT Mint Anticavity Fluoride Rinse	Sodium fluoride (0.02%)
CloSYS Fluoride Rinse	Sodium fluoride (0.05%)
Colgate Phos-Flur Ortho Defense (Bubblegum, Cool Mint, Gushing Grape flavors)	Sodium fluoride (0.05%)
Crest Anticavity Fluoride Rinse	Sodium fluoride (0.02%)
Crest Pro-Health Complete Rinse	Sodium fluoride (0.02%)
Firefly Anticavity Mouthrinse (Bubblegum, Strawberry, Melon flavors)	Sodium fluoride (0.05%)
Inspector Hector Tooth Protector Anticavity Rinse	Sodium fluoride (0.05%)
Kid's Crest Anticavity Fluoride Rinse	Sodium fluoride (0.02%)
Listerine Smart Rinse (Mint Shield, Berry Shield, Fab Bubble Gum, Bubble Blast flavors)	Sodium fluoride (0.02%)
Listerine Total Care Anticavity Mouthwash (Cinnamint, Fresh Mint flavors)	Sodium fluoride (0.02%)
Listerine Total Care Zero Anticavity Mouthwash	Sodium fluoride (0.02%)
The Natural Dentist Cavity Zapper Fluoride Rinse (Berry Blast flavor)	Sodium fluoride (0.05%)
Tom's of Maine Alcohol-free & Natural Children's Anticavity Fluoride Rinse (Juicy Mint flavor)	Sodium fluoride (0.05%)
Select store brands	Sodium fluoride (0.05%)

Table 2a. Anti-plaque/Gingivitis: Dentifrices

ADA SEAL ACCEPTED DENTIFRICES	ACTIVE INGREDIENTS
Colgate Total Advanced Deep Clean Toothpaste	Triclosan (0.30%)
Colgate Total Advanced Fresh + Whitening Gel	Triclosan (0.30%)
Colgate Total Clean Mint Toothpaste	Triclosan (0.30%)
Colgate Total Mint Stripe Toothpaste	Triclosan (0.30%)
Colgate Total Whitening Gel	Triclosan (0.30%)
Colgate Total Whitening Toothpaste	Triclosan (0.30%)
Crest Pro-Health Toothpaste (Cool Spearmint, Intense Peppermint flavors)	Stannous fluoride (0.454%)
Crest Pro-Health Advanced Deep Clean Mint Toothpaste	Stannous fluoride (0.454%)
Crest Pro-Health Extra Whitening Power	Stannous fluoride (0.454%)

Table 2b. Anti-plaque/Gingivitis: Mouthrinses

ADA SEAL ACCEPTED MOUTHRINSES	ACTIVE INGREDIENTS
Listerine Antiseptic (Original, Cool Mint, Fresh Burst, Soft Mint flavors)	Eucalyptol (0.092%), Menthol (0.042%), Methyl salicylate (0.060%), Thymol (0.064%)
Select store brands	Eucalyptol (0.092%), Menthol (0.042%), Methyl salicylate (0.060%), Thymol (0.064%)

Table 3. Hypersensitivity Management: Dentifrices

ADA SEAL ACCEPTED DENTIFRICES	ACTIVE INGREDIENTS
Sensodyne (Fresh Impact, Fresh Mint flavors)	Potassium nitrate (5%)
Crest Pro-Health Toothpaste (Cool Spearmint, Intense Peppermint flavors)	Stannous fluoride (0.454%)
Crest Pro-Health Advanced Deep Clean Mint Toothpaste	Stannous fluoride (0.454%)
Crest Pro-Health Extra Whitening Power	Stannous fluoride (0.454%)

Table 4. Prevention/Management of Erosion: Dentifrices

ADA SEAL ACCEPTED DENTIFRICES	ACTIVE INGREDIENTS
Crest Pro-Health Advanced Deep Clean Mint Toothpaste	Stannous fluoride (0.454%)

Table 5. Topical Oral Pain Relief Products

ADA SEAL ACCEPTED PRODUCTS	ACTIVE INGREDIENTS
Benzodent Dental Pain Relieving Cream	Benzocaine 20%
KANK-A MOUTH Pain Liquid Professional Strength	Benzocaine (20%), Compound Benzoin Tincture

Pediatric Drug
Management

Section 2:
Pediatric Drug Management

Martha Ann Keels, DDS, PhD and Erica Brecher, DMD, MS

1 | Analgesics Dosage

In order to alleviate pain in pediatric patients, systemic analgesics are indicated. Most commonly, acetaminophen or ibuprofen are utilized according to the dosing schedule below. For instances of moderate to severe pain, acetaminophen and ibuprofen can be alternated every three hours. The use of opioids for pain management in children is not recommended due to potential severe side effects.

Table 1. Pediatric Pain Medication		
Analgesic	**Sample Dosage**	**Forms**
Acetaminophen	10-15 mg/kg/dose given at 4-to 6- hour intervals	**Suspensions:** 160 mg/5 mL **Chewable Tablets:** 80 mg, 160 mg **Tablets:** 325 mg, 500 mg
Ibuprofen	4-10 mg/kg/dose given at 6- to 8-hour intervals	**Suspensions:** 100 mg/5 mL **Chewable Tablets:** 50 mg, 100 mg **Tablets:** 100 mg, 200 mg, (with prescription: 400, 600, and 800 mg)

2 | Anesthetic Dosage

To determine the local anesthetic dosage for a pediatric patient, one must determine the patient's weight pre-operatively. The potential for toxic reactions increases when local anesthetics are being combined with sedative medications. Therefore, when sedating a child, the local anesthetic dose needs to be adjusted downward. Moore and Hersh developed "The Rule of 25" as a simplified method for calculating the most conservative local anesthetic dose (see Suggested Reading list). The Rule of 25 states that for a healthy patient, a dentist can safely use 1 cartridge of anesthetic for every 25 pounds of weight. For example, a patient weighing 25 pounds could receive 1 carpule of anesthetic and a patient weighing 50 pounds could receive 2 carpules of anesthetic.

Phentolamine meslyalte (OraVerse) can be used in children over the age of six to reverse soft tissue anesthesia. The median lip recovery times were reduced by 75 to 85 minutes in clinical trials. Lingering numbness of the lower lip in pediatric patients can be a risk factor for self-inflicted mucosal trauma. The maximum recommended dose of Oraverse is ½ cartridge for children ages 6 to 11 weighing 33-66 pounds. One cartridge of OraVerse is recommended for children ages 6 to 11 weighing over 66 pounds.

Table 2. Anesthesia Dosages			
Anesthetics	**Maximum Dosage mg/kg, mg/lb**	**Maximum Total Dosage**	**Comments**
4% Articaine (1:100,000 epinephrine)	7.0 mg/kg 3.2 mg/lb	500 mg	Not recommended for use in children under 4 years
2% Lidocaine (1:100,000 epinephrine)	4.4 mg/kg 2.0 mg/lb	300 mg	
3% Mepivicaine (Plain)	4.4 mg/kg 2.0 mg/lb	300 mg	
4% Prilocaine (Plain or 1:200,000 epinephrine)	6.0 mg/kg 2.7 mg/lb	400 mg	Contraindicated in patients with methemoglobinemia, sickle cell anemia, or symptoms of hypoxia

3 | Antibiotic Use and Dosage

Three common areas where antibiotics may be indicated are with a) Odontogenic infections b) Infective endocarditis prophylaxis and c) Dental trauma. To avoid the development of resistant strains of bacteria, one must be prudent in prescribing antibiotics. Certain antibiotics, such as rifampicin, tetracycline, and penicillin derivatives can cause decreased plasma concentrations of oral contraceptives. Therefore, adolescent patients taking oral contraceptives will need to be advised to use additional precautions for contraception if given any of the described antibiotics.

3a | Odontogenic Infection Management

Antibiotics are not indicated if the child is afebrile or no facial swelling is present. Signs of systemic involvement such as fever or facial cellulitis warrant emergency management and administration of an oral antibiotic for 5 to 7 days. If the facial swelling is encroaching into the orbital space or the airway, then referral for medical management including intravenous antibiotics may be indicated.

Table 3. Antibiotics for Odontogenic Infections			
Antibiotic	**Sample Dosage**	**Forms**	**Comments**
Amoxicillin	**<40kg:** 20-40 mg/kg/day divided every 8 hr OR 25-45 mg/kg/day divided every 12 hr **>40kg:** 250-500 mg every 8 hr OR 500-875 mg every 12 hr	**Suspension:** 125 mg/5 mL, 250 mg/5 mL, 400 mg/5 mL **Chewable Tablet:** 125 mg, 250 mg **Tablet/Capsule:** 250 mg, 500 mg, 875 mg	Drug of choice for odontogenic infections
Amoxicillin/ Clavulanic Acid (Augmentin)*	**<40kg:** 25-45 mg/kg/day divided every 12 hr **>40kg:** 500-875 mg every 12 hr	**Suspension:** 125mg/31.25mg/5mL, 250mg/62.5mg/5mL, 400mg/57mg/5mL **Chewable Tablet:** 200mg/28.5mg, 400mg/57mg **Tablet/Capsule:** 250 mg/125 mg, 500 mg/125 mg, 875 mg/125 mg	Drug of choice for odontogenic infections with anaerobic bacterial involvement
Azithromycin	**<16 years:** 5-12 mg/kg once a day (maximum 500 mg/ day) **>16 years:** 250-600 mg once a day	**Suspension:** 100 mg/5 mL, 200 mg/5 mL, **Tablet/Capsule:** 250 mg, 500 mg	Alternative for type I allergy to penicillins/ cephalosporins
Clindamycin	**Children:** 8-20 mg/kg/day divided every 8 hr as hydrochloride salt OR 8-25 mg/kg/day divided every 8 hr as palmitate salt	**Suspension:** 75 mg/5 mL **Tablet/Capsule:** 150 mg, 300 mg	Alternative for type I allergy to penicillins/ cephalosporins Effective for infections with gram-positive aerobic bacteria and gram-positive or gram-negative anaerobic bacteria

* *Dosage Based on Amoxicillin Component.*

3b | Infective Endocarditis Prophylaxis

In 2007, the American Heart Association updated the guidelines for infective endocarditis prophylaxis. In particular, cardiac anomalies causing cyanosis require systemic antibiotic prophylaxis. However, one should refer to the most up-to-date version of the AHA guidelines to determine if the patient's cardiac condition requires antibiotic coverage. One should also consult the patient's cardiologist to verify the cardiac diagnosis and confirm the need for antibiotic coverage for specified dental procedures.

Table 4. Antibiotics for the Prevention of Infective Endocarditis Prophylaxis			
Antibiotic	Dosage	Forms	Comments
Amoxicillin	50 mg/kg ½ - 1 hr before dental procedure (maximum 2 g)	Refer to Table 3 Forms column	Drug of choice
Azithromycin	15 mg/kg ½ - 1 hr before dental procedure (maximum 500 mg)	Refer to Table 3 Forms column	Alternative for type I allergy to penicillins/ cephalosporins
Clindamycin	20 mg/kg ½ - 1 hr before dental procedure (maximum 600 mg)	Refer to Table 3 Forms column	Alternative for type I allergy to penicillins/ cephalosporins

3c | Dental Trauma

The benefit of administering a systemic antibiotic after replantation of an avulsed permanent incisor with open or closed apices is still questionable. However, experimental studies have shown promising results with both periodontal and pulpal healing after administering an antibiotic for 7 days. The first drug of choice is tetracycline. However, tetracycline is not recommended for children under the age of 12 due to the risk of intrinsic discoloration of the developing permanent teeth. Prior to age 12, amoxicillin can be given as an alternative medication to avoid the risk of discoloration of the permanent dentition.

Antibiotics are generally not indicated for luxation injuries in the primary or permanent dentitions.

Table 5. Antibiotics for Dental Trauma			
Antibiotic	**Sample Dosage**	**Forms**	**Comments**
Amoxicillin	**<40kg:** 20–40 mg/kg/day divided every 8h OR 25–45 mg/kg/day divided every 12 hr **>40kg:** 250–500 mg every 8 hr OR 500–875 mg every 12 hr	**Suspension:** 125 mg/5 mL, 250 mg/5 mL, 400 mg/5 mL **Chewable Tablet:** 125 mg, 250 mg **Tablet/Capsule:** 250 mg, 500 mg, 875 mg	Drug of choice for <12 years
Doxycycline	**<45 kg:** 2.2 mg/kg every 12 hr on day 1, then 2.2 mg/kg daily thereafter; for severe infections use 2.2 mg/kg every 12 hr **>45 kg:** 100 mg every 12 hr on day 1, then 100 mg daily thereafter, for severe infections use 100 mg every 12 hr	**Suspension:** 25 mg/5 mL **Tablet/Capsule:** 20 mg, 50 mg, 75 mg, 100 mg, 150 mg	Drug of choice for >12 years May cause permanent tooth discoloration, enamel hypoplasia in developing dentition.

4 | **Drugs to Avoid in Pediatrics**

Bupivacaine

This anesthetic is not recommended for children due to its long acting effect creating an increased risk of oral soft tissue trauma. One should also be cautious with administering viscous lidocaine to children for oral pain as children can be overly sensitive to this medication and overdose resulting in an acute breathing problem.

Codeine

With respect to pain management, children under 12 years should not take any medications that contain codeine. In addition, children between 12 and 18 years of age who are obese or having a pre-existing breathing problem should not be given codeine. Hence, Tylenol with codeine should not be used in children under 12 years of age.

Opioids

Recognizing the serious addiction potential with opioids, opioids are not recommended for pain management in children unless absolutely indicated. In these rare situations, dentists will need to follow the prescriptive guidelines for opioids recommended by their respective state dental board.

Tetracyclines

In addition to codeine, children under the age of 12 should not take tetracycline. It is well documented that consuming tetracycline prior to age 12 will cause intrinsic staining of the dentin in any developing permanent tooth at the time of drug administration. After age 12, the large majority of the permanent teeth have calcified and are no longer at risk of intrinsic color changes.

5 ｜ Drugs Recommended in Emergencies

In the unfortunate event that a pediatric medical emergency arises, the following medications should be available on hand in any dental practice. Listed below in Table 6 are the medications needed to assist in the management of the most common pediatric dental emergencies. Additional medications may be required by individual dental state boards.

Table 6. Pediatric Emergency Drugs				
Drug	Indication	Mechanism of Action	Sample Dosage	Delivery System
Albuterol	Acute asthma	B2 Agonist	1-2 inhalations	Inhaled
Diazepam	Status epilepticus	Anticonvulsant	<5 years: 5 mg >5 years: 10 mg	Rectal
Diphenhydramine	Mild allergic reaction (hives, itching, edema)	Histamine-1 receptor agonist	1 mg/kg	Oral
Epinephrine	Severe allergic reaction (anaphylaxis, acute asthma)	Sympathomimetic	0.01 mg/kg 1:1000 every 5 min or Autoinjector: 0.15 mg or 0.3 mg	SubQ, IM IM
Flumazenil	Benzodiazepine reversal	GABA receptor antagonist	0.01 mg/kg every 1 min (maximum 0.2 mg)	IM, IV
Glucose	Hypoglycemia conscious patient	Increased blood sugar	Gel, frosting, juice	Oral
Naloxone	Opioid reversal	Opioid receptor antagonist	0.1 mg/kg every 2-3 min (maximum 2 mg)	SubQ, IM, IV

📖 | **Suggested Reading**

- Malamed SF. Anesthetic considerations in dental specialities. In: Handbook of Local Anesthesia. 6th ed. St. Loius, Mo: Mosby; 2013: 277-89.

- Dean JA, Avery DR, McDonald RE. Local anesthesia for the child and adolescent. In: Dentistry for the Child and Adolescent. 10th ed., St Loius, Mo.: Mosby; 2016: 274-85.

- Moore PA, Hersh EV: Local anesthetics: pharmacology and toxicology, Dental Clin North Am 2010; 54:587-99.

- Wilson W, Taubert KA, Gevitz M, et al. Prevention of infective endocariditis: Guidelines from the American Heart Association; Circulation 2007; 116 (15): 1736-54. Erratum in Circulation 2007; 116 (15): e376-e7.

- Andersson l, Andreasen JO, Day P, et al. Guidelines for the Management of Traumatic Injuries. 2. Avulsion of Permanent Teeth. Dental Traumatology 2012; 28:88-96.

- Tate AR, Acs G: Dental postoperative pain management in children. Dental Clin North Am 2002; 46: 707-717.

- Tobias JD, Green TP, Cote CJ, Section on Anesthesiology and Pain Medicine, Committee on Drugs. : Codeine: Time to Say "No". *http://pediatrics.aappublications.org/content/early/2016/09/15/peds.2016-2396.*

Emergency Drug
Management

Section 3:
Emergency Drug Management

Jay Elkareh, PharmD, PhD

1 | Emergency Preparedness

Medical emergencies can occur in the dental office. Malamed found that 96.6% of dentists reported experiencing a medical emergency in the dental office at some point. Syncope and mild allergic reactions represent almost 50% of medical emergencies in a study he cites that involved 2,704 dentists (see Suggested Reading List).

One of the worst medical emergencies to be faced with is cardiac arrest. One study reported 148 cardiac arrests experienced in the offices of 2,704 dentists within a 10-year period (see Malamed, Suggested Reading List). For this reason, all personnel in a dental office should be trained in basic life support.

A good approach to emergency preparedness is to assign each dental professional a specific responsibility that may be needed during an emergent situation. For example, you would have an emergency team leader take care of the patient, including tasks such as:

- positioning the patient in a chair
- performing airway, breathing, and circulation assessments
- administering the appropriate medications
- performing CPR, if necessary

The emergency team leader has to appear calm and collected and stay with the patient at all times.

The critical care medical assistant will handle the supplies and medications, including tasks such as:

- bringing the emergency kit
- preparing the medication for administration
- providing oxygen via the defined delivery system
- monitoring the vital signs
- bringing the defibrillator
- assisting in the CPR process, when necessary

The critical care medical assistant also will act as a team lead in the absence of the team lead. The critical care medical assistant has to restock the medications and supplies used during the process, and is responsible for checking both the oxygen tank level and the medication expiration dates on a monthly basis.

Finally, the critical care coordinator will be in charge of coordinating calls and documentation, including tasks such as:

- calling EMS (911)
- meeting the paramedics
- keeping chronological records of all vital signs, medication doses and patient's response to treatment

The critical care coordinator will act as an emergency team assistant or as a team lead, if needed.

In summary:

- **Emergency Team Leader** takes care of the patient, and stays with the patient at all times.
- **Critical Care Medical Assistant** takes care of the equipment, the medication, and the supplies.
- **Critical Care Coordinator** takes care of the documentation, and the coordination with the emergency medical services.

2 | Emergency Drugs

The ADA Council on Scientific Affairs stated the following in a 2002 report in the *Journal of the American Dental Association*, Volume 133, No 3, 364–365 titled "Office Emergencies and Emergency Kits":

"In designing an emergency drug kit, the Council suggests that the following drugs be included as a minimum: epinephrine 1:1,000 (injectable), histamine-blocker (injectable), oxygen with positive-pressure administration capability, nitroglycerin (sublingual tablet or aerosol spray), bronchodilator (asthma inhaler), sugar and aspirin. Other drugs may be included as the doctor's training and needs mandate. It is particularly important that the dentist be knowledgeable about the indications, contraindications, dosages and methods of delivery for all items included in the emergency kit. Dentists are also urged to perform continual emergency kit maintenance by replacing soon-to-be-outdated drugs before their expiration."

The flow chart provides a suggested list of the basic emergency drugs that should be present in every dental office for various emergency situations. The choice of drug, its administration and expected effects depend on the symptoms experienced by the patient. The critical care team should monitor vital signs and call the EMS/911 when drug administration fails or symptoms worsen. In addition, medication and equipment must be checked on a monthly basis to ensure that it will be ready to use in an emergency.

Many states also require dental offices to have certain emergency drugs and equipment and most importantly to be prepared for emergency events through certifications and training. For additional information about the safety requirements in your state, consult with your state dental association or your state board of dental practice.

Tables 1a-j | Medication Options for Medical Emergencies

Table 1a. Allergic Reaction	
Symptoms	• Rash, urticaria, with no evidence of airway obstruction
Drug to Use	• Diphenhydramine 50 mg/mL
How to Use	• Adults: 50 mg by mouth/1 mL IM • Children: 25 mg by mouth/0.5 mL IM
Expected Effects	• Onset of action 15-30 min for by mouth, and <10 min for IM, • Reduction in pruritic, and cholinergic symptoms • Sedation, hypotension
Monitor or Avoid	None
What to do next	• If symptoms do not resolve and/or laryngeal edema is suspected, use epinephrine 1 mg/mL, 0.3 mL IM for adults and 0.15 mL IM for children

Table 1b. Anaphylaxis		
Symptoms	• Rash, urticaria, tongue or throat swelling	
Drug to Use	• Epinephrine 1 mg/mL	• Hydrocortisone sodium succinate 100 mg to dissolve in 2 mL bacteriostatic water	• Diphenhydramine 50 mg/mL
How to Use	• Adults: 0.3 mL IM • Children: 0.15 mL IM • 1 mL IV every 5 min • Can repeat once more as needed	• Adults: 2 mL IM or IV • Children: 2mg/kg/ dose IM • Can repeat 3 times as needed every 2 hrs	• Adults: 50 mg by mouth/1 mL IM • Children: 25 mg by mouth/0.5 mL IM
Expected Effects	• Increase in heart rate • Decrease in allergic reaction	• Nervousness, irritation • Decrease in allergic reaction	• Reduction in pruritic and cholinergic symptoms • Sedation, hypotension
Monitor or Avoid	• Monitor vital signs at all times		
What to do next	• If symptoms do not resolve after 2 doses of Epinephrine, call EMS/911		

Table 1c. Asthmatic Reaction	
Symptoms	• Shortness of breath or difficulty breathing with no swelling in the throat
Drug to Use	• Albuterol 90 mcg inhaler
How to Use	• 2-3 puffs inhalation every 1-2 min • Repeat 3 times as needed
Expected Effects	• Increase in oxygen levels • Reduction in airway resistance • Tachycardia, hypertension, restlessness, nervousness
Monitor or Avoid	• Monitor vital signs at all times • Consider using oxygen, especially when the O_2 saturation starts dropping
What to do next	• If symptoms do not resolve, use methylprednisolone 80 mg/mL, 3 mL intramuscularly as a one-time dose • If symptoms do not resolve, and/or laryngeal edema is suspected, use epinephrine

Table 1d. Benzodiazepine and Z-drugs Intoxication	
Symptoms	• Deep sedation, blurred vision, slow labored breathing
Drug to Use	• Flumazenil 0.1 mg/mL (reversal drug)
How to Use	• Inject 2 mL sublingual Q3-5 min • Repeat up to 4 times as needed due to its short duration of action <1 hr
Expected Effects	• Reverse in sedative effects • Agitation, anxiety, panic attacks, seizure • Arrhythmia
Monitor or Avoid	• Don't use in patients chronically on benzodiazepines or Z-drugs (such as Ambien, Lunesta, Sonata) unless life threatening
What to do next	• If symptoms do not resolve after 4 doses of Flumazenil, call EMS • Keep the patient calm, and continue oxygen supply until EMS arrival

Table 1e. Chest Pain (Angina)

Symptoms	• Sharp and sudden pain in the chest, the jaw or the neck • Chest pain could be the result of gastroesophageal reflux or anxiety attack, but angina treatment trumps the latter two symptoms		
Drug to Use	• Nitroglycerin 0.4 mg	• Aspirin 325 mg	• Morphine 1 mg/mL*
How to Use	• 1 tablet sublingual every 5 min • Repeat 2 times as needed while awaiting for emergency medical services (EMS)	• 1 enteric coated tablet to chew and swallow	• Only use if pain is acute and not resolved by nitroglycerin • 2 to 4 mL IV push every 5 to 15 min as needed for pain
Expected Effects	• Reduction in myocardial oxygen demand • Flushing in face and neck • Headache, and orthostatic hypotension	• Decrease platelet aggregation and prevent clot formation	• Reduction in pain and anxiety • Reduction in blood pressure • Respiratory depression
Monitor or Avoid	• Monitor vital signs at all times		
What to do next	• If symptoms do not resolve after 1 dose of nitroglycerin, call EMS/911 • Repeat nitroglycerin administration up to x2 while waiting for EMS/911		

* When morphine is used oxygen therapy should be administered simultaneously especially when the pulse oximeter oxygen saturation SpO$_2$ reads or falls below 94%. MONA therapy (Morphine, Oxygen, Nitroglycerin, Aspirin) is implemented in this case.

Table 1f. Hypoglycemia

Symptoms	• Tachycardia, shakiness and excessive sweating
Drug to Use	• Viscous glucose concentrate (Instaglucose gel 31 g)
How to Use	• Squirt ½ tube in mouth
Expected Effects	• Smooth muscle relaxation and reduction in hypoglycemic symptoms
Monitor or Avoid	None
What to do next	N/A

Table 1g. Hypotension

	without bradycardia	with bradycardia
Symptoms	• lightheadedness, blurred vision, clammy skin	• lightheadedness, blurred vision, clammy skin
Drug to Use	• Ephedrine 50 mg/mL	• Atropine 1 mg/mL • More powerful and shorter duration of action than ephedrine
How to Use	• Inject 0.5 mL SL or IM every 5 min • Can repeat once more as needed	• Inject 0.5 mL SL or IM every 5 min • Can repeat 5 times as needed
Expected Effects	• Increase in heart rate • Increase in blood pressure	• Increase in heart rate • Increase in blood pressure
Monitor or Avoid	• Monitor vital signs at all times	• Monitor vital signs at all times
What to do next	• If symptoms do not resolve after 2 doses use atropine	• If symptoms do not resolve after 2 doses, call EMS/911 • Repeat drug administration up to x5 while waiting for EMS/911

Table 1h. Opioids Intoxication	
Symptoms	• Delirium, pinpoint pupils, slow irregular breathing, cold skin with bluish lips and fingernails
Drug to Use	• Naloxone 0.4 mg/mL (reversal drug)
How to Use	• Inject 1 mL SL every 3-5 min • Advise to repeat once more as needed due to its short duration of action
Expected Effects	• Reverse in sedative effects • Increases respiratory rate • Increases blood pressure
Monitor or Avoid	• Monitor vital signs at all times • Don't use in patients who are opioid dependent to avoid withdrawal symptoms, unless life threatening
What to do next	• If symptoms do not resolve after 2 doses of Naloxone, call EMS, • Keep the patient calm, and continue oxygen supply until EMS arrival

Table 1i. Seizure	
Symptoms	• Rhythmic muscle contractions or muscle spasms, temporary paralysis, loss of consciousness
Drug to Use	• Lorazepam 2 mg/mL
How to Use	• Inject 2 mL intravenously over 2 minutes (dilute in saline 1:1 ratio) • May repeat once more as needed in 5-10 min
Expected Effects	• Muscle relaxation • Decreased nervousness • Orthostatic hypotension
Monitor or Avoid	• Monitor vital signs at all times
What to do next	• If symptoms do not resolve after 2 doses of Lorazepam, call EMS • Keep the patient calm, and continue oxygen supply until EMS arrival

Table 1j. Syncope	
Symptoms	• Pale skin, cold sweat, lightheadedness, and heaviness in the legs
Drug to Use	• Aromatic ammonia
How to Use	• Crush ampule and hold 4-6 inches under the nose
Expected Effects	• Respiratory stimulant • Coughing, watery eyes
Monitor or Avoid	None
What to do next	• Consider using oxygen to improve oxygenation of peripheral tissues if symptoms don't resolve

📖 | Suggested Reading

- Boyd BC, Hall RE. Drugs for medical emergencies in the dental office. Ciancio S, ed. ADA/PDR Guide to dental therapeutics. Fifth ed. Chicago: American Dental Association, 2009.

- Becker DE. Emergency drug kits: pharmacological and technical considerations. Anesth Prog 2014;61(4):171-9.

- Dym H, Barzani G, Mohan N. Emergency drugs for the dental office. Dent Clin North Am 2016;60(2):287-94.

- Haas DA. Preparing dental office staff members for emergencies: developing a basic action plan. J Am Dent Assoc 2010;141 Suppl 1:8s-13s.

- Malamed SF. Knowing your patients. J Am Dent Assoc 2010;141 Suppl 1:3s-7s.

- Rosenberg M, Preparing for Medical Emergencies J Am Dent Assoc 2010;141, Supplement 1, Pages S14–S19

Special Care
Patients

- Guidelines in Specific Procedures
- Guidance in Specific Populations

Section 4:
Guidelines in Specific Procedures: Antibiotic Prophylaxis, MRONJ, Sedation and General Anesthesia

Prepared by Kathleen Ziegler, PharmD

Antibiotic Prophylaxis Prior to Dental Procedures

Among some patients, there are formal recommendations. Recommendations for antibiotic prophylaxis prior to certain dental procedures exist primarily for two groups:

- patients with heart conditions that may predispose them to infective endocarditis; and
- patients who have a prosthetic joint(s) and may be at risk for developing hematogenous infections at the site of the prosthetic.

However, compared with earlier iterations, the current recommendations identify relatively few patient subpopulations within these groups for whom antibiotic prophylaxis may be indicated.

1 | Prevention of Prosthetic Joint Infection

In 2014, the ADA Council on Scientific Affairs assembled an expert panel to update and clarify the clinical recommendations found in the 2012 evidence report and 2013 guideline: Prevention of Orthopaedic Implant Infection in Patients Undergoing Dental Procedures (see Suggested Reading List).

As was found in 2012, the updated systematic review published in 2015 found no association between dental procedures and prosthetic joint infections. Based on this evidence review, the 2015 ADA clinical practice guideline states, "In general, for patients with prosthetic joint implants, prophylactic antibiotics are not recommended prior to dental procedures to prevent prosthetic joint infection."

In 2017, an ADA-appointed panel of experts published a commentary in *JADA* (see Suggested Reading List), offering guidance for using the American Academy of Orthopaedic Surgeons' "appropriate use criteria," which address managing care for patients with orthopedic implants undergoing dental procedures (see Suggested Reading List). The JADA piece calls the appropriate use criteria "a decision-support tool to supplement clinicians in their judgment" and it emphasizes discussion of available treatment options between the patient, dentist and orthopedic surgeon, weighing the potential risks and benefits. The commentary encourages dentists to continue to use the 2015 guideline, consult the appropriate use criteria as needed, and respect the patient's specific needs and preferences when considering antibiotic prophylaxis before dental treatment.

According to the ADA Chairside Guide developed by the Center for Evidence-based Dentistry (see Suggested Reading List), "for patients with a history of complications associated with their joint replacement surgery who are undergoing dental procedures that include gingival manipulation or mucosal incision, prophylactic antibiotics should only be considered after consultation with the patient and orthopedic surgeon." Further, in cases where antibiotics are deemed necessary, it is most appropriate that the orthopedic surgeon recommend the antibiotic regimen and, when reasonable, write the prescription.

2 | Prevention of Infective Endocarditis

With input from the ADA, the American Heart Association (AHA) released guidelines for the prevention of infective endocarditis in 2007, which were approved by the CSA as they relate to dentistry in 2008. In 2017, the AHA and American College of Cardiology (ACC) published a focused update to their 2014 guidelines on the management of valvular heart disease that reinforce the previous recommendations.

These current guidelines support infective endocarditis premedication for a relatively small subset of patients. This is based on a review of scientific evidence, which showed that the risk of adverse reactions to antibiotics generally outweigh the benefits of prophylaxis for many patients who would have been considered eligible for prophylaxis in previous versions of the guidelines. Concern about the development of drug-resistant bacteria also was a factor.

Also, the data are inconsistent as to whether prophylactic antibiotics taken before a dental procedure prevent infective endocarditis. The guidelines note that people who are at risk for infective endocarditis are regularly exposed to oral bacteria during basic daily activities such as brushing or flossing.

The valvular disease management guidelines recommend that persons at risk of developing bacterial infective endocarditis (Box 1) establish and maintain the best possible oral health to reduce potential sources of bacterial seeding. They state, "Optimal oral health is maintained through regular professional dental care and the use of appropriate dental products, such as manual, powered, and ultrasonic toothbrushes; dental floss; and other plaque-removal devices."

3 | Dental Procedures

Prophylaxis is recommended for the patients identified in the previous section for all dental procedures that involve manipulation of gingival tissue or the periapical region of the teeth, or perforation of the oral mucosa. Refer to Antibiotics chapter (Chapter 2) for more information.

Box 1. Patient Selection for Persons at Risk of Developing Bacterial Infective Endocarditis

The current infective endocarditis/valvular heart disease guidelines state that use of preventive antibiotics before certain dental procedures is reasonable for patients with:

- prosthetic cardiac valves, including transcatheter-implanted prostheses and homografts
- prosthetic material used for cardiac valve repair, such as annuloplasty rings and chords
- a history of infective endocarditis
- a cardiac transplant* with valve regurgitation due to a structurally abnormal valve;
- the following congenital (present from birth) heart disease:**
  - unrepaired cyanotic congenital heart disease, including palliative shunts and conduits
  - any repaired congenital heart defect with residual shunts or valvular regurgitation at the site of or adjacent to the site of a prosthetic patch or a prosthetic device

* According to limited data, infective endocarditis appears to be more common in heart transplant recipients than in the general population; the risk of infective endocarditis is highest in the first 6 months after transplant because of endothelial disruption, high-intensity immunosuppressive therapy, frequent central venous catheter access, and frequent endomyocardial biopsies.

** Except for the conditions listed above, antibiotic prophylaxis is not recommended for any other form of congenital heart disease.

📖 | Suggested Reading

- American Academy of Orthopaedic Surgeons. Appropriate Use Criteria: Management of Patients with Orthopaedic Implants Undergoing Dental Procedures. *https://aaos. webauthor.com/go/auc/terms.cfm?auc_id=224995&actionxm=Terms*. Accessed August 3, 2018.
- American Academy of Orthopaedic Surgeons; American Dental Association. Prevention of orthopaedic implant infection in patients undergoing dental procedures: evidence-based guideline and evidence report. Rosemont, IL: American Academy of Orthopaedic Surgeons; 2012. Available at: *https://www.aaos.org/ Research/guidelines/PUDP/PUDP_guideline.pdf*. Accessed August 3, 2018.
- American Dental Association-Appointed Members of the Expert Writing and Voting Panels Contributing to the Development of American Academy of Orthopedic Surgeons Appropriate Use Criteria. American Dental Association guidance for utilizing appropriate use criteria in the management of the care of patients with orthopedic implants undergoing dental procedures. J Am Dent Assoc 2017;148(2):57-59.
- American Dental Association Center for Evidence-Based Dentistry. Chairside Guide, 2015. *https://ebd.ada.org/~/media/EBD/Images/Chairside%20Guides/ADA_ Chairside_Guide_Prosthetics.pdf?la=en*.
- Meyer DM. Providing clarity on evidence-based prophylactic guidelines for prosthetic joint infections. J Am Dent Assoc 2015;146(1):3-5.

- Sollecito TP, Abt E, Lockhart PB, et al. The use of prophylactic antibiotics prior to dental procedures in patients with prosthetic joints: Evidence-based clinical practice guideline for dental practitioners--a report of the American Dental Association Council on Scientific Affairs. J Am Dent Assoc 2015;146(1):11-16 e8.

- Wilson W, Taubert KA, Gewitz M, et al. Prevention of infective endocarditis: guidelines from the American Heart Association: a guideline from the American Heart Association Rheumatic Fever, Endocarditis, and Kawasaki Disease Committee, Council on Cardiovascular Disease in the Young, and the Council on Clinical Cardiology, Council on Cardiovascular Surgery and Anesthesia, and the Quality of Care and Outcomes Research Interdisciplinary Working Group. Circulation 2007;116(15):1736-54.

- Wilson W, Taubert KA, Gewitz M, et al. Prevention of infective endocarditis: guidelines from the American Heart Association: a guideline from the American Heart Association Rheumatic Fever, Endocarditis and Kawasaki Disease Committee, Council on Cardiovascular Disease in the Young, and the Council on Clinical Cardiology, Council on Cardiovascular Surgery and Anesthesia, and the Quality of Care and Outcomes Research Interdisciplinary Working Group. J Am Dent Assoc 2008;139 Suppl:3S-24S.

Medication-Related Osteonecrosis of the Jaw

In 2014, the American Association of Oral and Maxillofacial Surgeons (AAOMS) updated their definition of Medication-Related Osteonecrosis of the Jaw (MRONJ) (see Ruggiero et al in Suggested Reading List) to include all of the following criteria: (1) current or previous treatment with antiresorptive or antiangiogenic agents; (2) exposed bone or bone that can be probed through an intraoral or extraoral fistula(e) in the maxillofacial region that has persisted for more than 8 weeks; and (3) no history of radiation therapy to the jaws or obvious metastatic disease to the jaws.

The reported incidence of MRONJ varies, but it is generally considered to be between 1% and 10% of patients taking IV bisphosphonates for the management of bone metastatic disease and between 0.001% and 0.01% in patients taking oral bisphosphonates for the management of osteoporosis.

The differential diagnosis of MRONJ includes other conditions such as alveolar osteitis, sinusitis, gingivitis/periodontitis, or periapical pathosis. According to a 2015 systematic review and international consensus paper by Khan et al. (see Suggested Reading List), patient history and clinical examination remain the most sensitive diagnostic tools for MRONJ. While it is not possible to identify who will develop MRONJ and who will not, research suggests the following as risk factors:

- age older than 65 years
- periodontitis
- recent dentoalveolar surgery, including tooth extraction
- high dose and/or prolonged use of antiresorptive agents (i.e., more than 2 years)
- receiving antiresorptive therapy in conjunction with antiangiogenic drugs for cancer
- smoking
- malignant disease (multiple myeloma, and breast, prostate, and lung cancer)
- chemotherapy, corticosteroid therapy, or treatment with antiangiogenic agents
- denture wearing
- diabetes

1 | Dental Patients Receiving Antiresorptive Medications for Osteoporosis

In November 2011, the ADA Council on Scientific Affairs (CSA) Expert Panel on Antiresorptive Agents published recommendations for managing the dental care of patients receiving antiresorptive therapy specifically for the prevention and treatment of osteoporosis (i.e., not addressing the dental care of patients being treated with antiresorptive agents as part of cancer therapy)(see Suggested Reading List). These recommendations were based on a narrative review of the literature from May 2008 (the date of the last search for a 2008 review and statement) through February 2011.

Although the 2008 report limited the review to jaw osteonecrosis related to bisphosphonates, the 2011 report expanded the search to include jaw osteonecrosis related to the use of any antiresorptive agent (including denosumab and cathepsin K inhibitors).

The CSA report found that the highest reliable estimate of MRONJ prevalence is low (approximately 0.10%) in patients receiving drug dosages and regimens intended to treat or prevent osteoporosis. The CSA concluded that the potential morbidity and mortality associated with osteoporosis-related fracture is considerable and treatment with antiresorptive agents, including bisphosphonates, outweighs the low risk of MRONJ in patients with osteoporosis being treated with these drugs. The report states that "An oral health program consisting of sound hygiene practices and regular dental care may be the optimal approach for lowering [MRONJ] risk" in these patients and that a discussion of the risks and benefits of dental care with patients receiving antiresorptive therapy is appropriate. The report provides the following points that dental practitioners can discuss with patients:

- Antiresorptive therapy for low bone mass places patients at a low risk of developing drug-related ONJ
- The low risk of MRONJ can be reduced, but not eliminated
- An oral health program consisting of sound oral hygiene practices and regular dental care may lower the risk of drug-related ONJ
- As of this writing, no validated prognostic tool is available to determine which patients are at increased risk of developing drug-related ONJ
- Due to the cumulative effect of bisphosphonates in the bone, discontinuing bisphosphonate therapy may not eliminate the risk of developing drug-related ONJ and that discontinuation of bisphosphonate therapy may have a negative impact on the outcomes of treatment for low bone mass

Because of the paucity of clinical data regarding the dental care of patients receiving antiresorptive therapy, the report also describes management recommendations based primarily on expert opinion for general prevention and treatment planning, as well as for specific conditions, such as management of periodontal disease, oral and maxillofacial surgery, endodontics, restorative dentistry and prosthodontics, and orthodontics (Table 1). There is insufficient evidence to recommend a "holiday" from antiresorptive drug therapy for osteoporosis or waiting periods before performing dental treatment for prevention of MRONJ. There is also insufficient evidence to recommend the use of serum biomarker tests, such as serum C-terminal telopeptide (CTX) as a predictor of MRONJ risk in patients receiving the drugs for osteoporosis indications.

Table 1. Dental Intervention and Recommendations for Dental Patients Receiving Antiresorptive Therapy Based on Expert Opinion*
General Prevention and Treatment Planning:
<ul><li>Have a discussion with patients regarding potential risks and benefits</li><li>Do not modify routine dental treatment solely because of osteoporosis antiresorptive medications</li><li>A localized clinical approach (e.g., treating a sextant at a time) to dentoalveolar surgery in patients receiving antiresorptive therapy for low bone density may help assess risk (Note, the sextant-by-sextant approach does not apply to emergency cases, even if multiple quadrants are involved)</li><li>Treat periapical pathoses, sinus tracts, purulent periodontal pockets, severe periodontitis and active abscesses that already involve the medullary bone expeditiously</li></ul>

Management of Periodontal Disease:

- Obtain access to root surfaces using atraumatic techniques that minimize dentoalveolar manipulation whenever possible
- Use techniques such as guided tissue regeneration or bone grafting judiciously based on patient need
- Primary soft-tissue closure after periodontal surgical procedures is desirable, when feasible, although extended periosteal bone exposure for the sake of primary closure may increase, rather than decrease, the risk of developing MRONJ

Implant Placement and Maintenance:

- Antiresorptive therapy does not appear to be a contraindication for dental implant placement; however, larger and longer-term studies are needed to determine if implants placed in patients exposed to antiresorptive agents perform as well as those placed in patients who have not been exposed to these agents

Oral and Maxillofacial Surgery:

- If extractions or bone surgery is necessary, dentists should consider a conservative surgical technique with primary tissue closure, when feasible
- Placement of semipermeable membranes over extraction sites also may be appropriate if primary closure is not possible
- Before and after any surgical procedures involving bone, the patient should rinse gently with a chlorhexidine-containing rinse until the extraction site has healed

Endodontics:

- In patients with an elevated risk of developing MRONJ, endodontic treatment is preferable to surgical manipulation if a tooth is salvageable
- Practitioners should use a routine endodontic technique; however, the panel does not recommend manipulation beyond the apex

Restorative Dentistry and Prosthodontics:

- Practitioners should perform all routine restorative procedures with the goal of minimizing the impact on bone, so as not to increase the risk of infection
- To avoid ulceration and possible bone exposure, practitioners should adjust prosthodontic appliances promptly for fit

Orthodontics:

- Inhibited tooth movement in adult patients receiving bisphosphonate therapy has been reported and dentists should advise patients of this potential complication; however, orthodontic procedures have been performed successfully in patients receiving antiresorptive therapy, and it is not necessarily contraindicated
- Orthognathic surgery and tooth extractions result in more extensive bone healing and remodeling; treatment planning in these cases may require increased vigilance

* Hellstein JW, Adler RA, Edwards B, et al. Managing the care of patients receiving antiresorptive therapy for prevention and treatment of osteoporosis: Recommendations from the American Dental Association Council on Scientific Affairs (Narrative review). November 2011. (*https://www.aae. org/uploadedfiles/publications_and_research/endodontics_colleagues_for_excellence_newsletter/ bonj_ada_report.pdf*. Accessed August 3, 2018.)

2 | Dental Patients Receiving Antiresorptive or Antiangiogenic Medications for Cancer

In 2014, AAOMS published a position paper on MRONJ (see Ruggiero et al., Suggested Reading List). The position paper was based on a literature review and expert opinion/observations of a multidisciplinary committee including surgeons, pathologists, and oncologists. Although the authors cautioned that the position paper was informational in nature and not intended to set any standards of care, they did provide suggestions for potential prevention strategies for patients based on limited evidence, including implementation of dental screening and appropriate dental interventions before initiating antiresorptive and/or antiangiogenic therapies. In patients receiving antiresorptive and/or antiangiogenic medications for cancer-related indications, increased awareness, preventive dental care, and early recognition of the signs and symptoms of MRONJ may result in earlier detection.

The AAOMS committee outlined the following measures as part of early treatment planning in these patients:

- thorough examination of the oral cavity and a radiographic assessment when indicated
- identification of acute infection and sites of potential infection to prevent future sequelae that could be exacerbated once drug therapy begins
- patient motivation and patient education regarding dental care

The AAOMS article by Ruggiero et al. states that if "systemic conditions permit, initiation of antiresorptive therapy should be delayed until dental health is optimized" and that "This decision must be made in conjunction with the treating physician and dentist and other specialists involved in the care of the patient" (see Suggested Reading List) Regarding antiangiogenic therapy, the AAOMS states, "There are no data to support or refute the cessation of antiangiogenic therapy in the prevention or management of MRONJ; therefore, continued research in the area is indicated."

A systematic review and international consensus paper from the International Task Force on Osteonecrosis of the Jaw published in early 2015 also suggests that key prevention strategies for MRONJ include elimination or stabilization of oral disease prior to initiation of antiresorptive agents, as well as maintenance of good oral hygiene (See Khan, Suggested Reading List). For patients whose cancer management includes treatment with denosumab or IV bisphosphonates, the Task Force recommends that "a thorough dental examination with dental radiographs should be ideally completed prior to the initiation of antiresorptive therapy in order to identify dental disease before drug therapy is initiated" and that "Any necessary invasive dental procedure including dental extractions or implants should ideally be completed prior to initiation of [bisphosphonate] or [denosumab] therapy."

The Task Force also states that, "Non-urgent procedures should be assessed for optimal timing because it may be appropriate to complete the non-urgent procedure prior to osteoclast inhibition, delay it until it is necessary, or perhaps plan for it during a drug holiday; however, there are no compelling data to guide these decisions."

📖 | **Suggested Reading**

- Beth-Tasdogan NH, Mayer B, Hussein H, Zolk O. Interventions for managing medication-related osteonecrosis of the jaw. Cochrane Database Syst Rev 2017;10:Cd012432.

- Hellstein JW, Adler RA, Edwards B, et al. Managing the care of patients receiving antiresorptive therapy for prevention and treatment of osteoporosis: Recommendations from the American Dental Association Council on Scientific Affairs (Narrative review). November 2011. *https://www.aae.org/uploadedfiles/publications_and_research/endodontics_colleagues_for_excellence_newsletter/bonj_ada_report.pdf.*

- Hellstein JW, Adler RA, Edwards B, et al. Managing the care of patients receiving antiresorptive therapy for prevention and treatment of osteoporosis: executive summary of recommendations from the American Dental Association Council on Scientific Affairs. J Am Dent Assoc 2011;142(11):1243-51.

- Khan AA, Morrison A, Hanley DA, et al. Diagnosis and management of osteonecrosis of the jaw: a systematic review and international consensus. J Bone Miner Res 2015;30(1):3-23.

- No Authors Listed. Osteoporosis medications and your dental health. J Am Dent Assoc 2011;142(11):1320.

- Ruggiero SL, Dodson TB, Fantasia J, et al. American Association of Oral and Maxillofacial Surgeons position paper on medication-related osteonecrosis of the jaw--2014 update. J Oral Maxillofac Surg 2014;72(10):1938-56.

- Yamashita J, McCauley LK. Antiresorptives and osteonecrosis of the jaw. J Evid Based Dent Pract 2012;12(3 Suppl):233-47.

Sedation and General Anesthesia Guidelines

Excerpted from: American Dental Association. ADA Guidelines for the Use of Sedation and General Anesthesia by Dentists, October 2016.

http://www.ada.org/~/media/ADA/Education%20and%20Careers/Files/ADA_Sedation_Use_Guidelines.pdf?la=en

The administration of local anesthesia, sedation and general anesthesia is an integral part of dental practice. The American Dental Association is committed to the safe and effective use of these modalities by appropriately educated and trained dentists. The purpose of these guidelines is to assist dentists in the delivery of safe and effective sedation and anesthesia (Box 2).

Dentists must comply with their state laws, rules and/or regulations when providing sedation and anesthesia

Level of sedation is entirely independent of the route of administration. Moderate and deep sedation or general anesthesia may be achieved via any route of administration and thus an appropriately consistent level of training must be established.

For children, the American Dental Association supports the use of the American Academy of Pediatrics/American Academy of Pediatric Dentistry Guidelines for Monitoring and Management of Pediatric Patients During and After Sedation for Diagnostic and Therapeutic Procedures.

Box 2. Clinical Guidelines[1]*

A. Minimal Sedation

1. **Patient History and Evaluation**

   Patients considered for minimal sedation must be suitably evaluated prior to the start of any sedative procedure. In healthy or medically stable individuals (ASA I, II)[2] this should consist of a review of their current medical history and medication use. In addition, patients with significant medical considerations (ASA III, IV)[2] may require consultation with their primary care physician or consulting medical specialist.

2. **Preoperative Evaluation and Preparation**

   - The patient, parent, legal guardian or care giver must be advised regarding the procedure associated with the delivery of any sedative agents and informed consent for the proposed sedation must be obtained.
   - Determination of adequate oxygen supply and equipment necessary to deliver oxygen under positive pressure must be completed.
   - An appropriate focused physical evaluation should be performed.
   - Baseline vital signs including body weight, height, blood pressure, pulse rate, and respiration rate must be obtained unless invalidated by the nature of the patient, procedure or equipment. Body temperature should be measured when clinically indicated.
   - Preoperative dietary restrictions must be considered based on the sedative technique prescribed.
   - Preoperative verbal and written instructions must be given to the patient, parent, escort, legal guardian or caregiver.

3. **Personnel and Equipment Requirements**

   Personnel: At least one additional person trained in Basic Life Support for Healthcare Providers must be present in addition to the dentist.

   Equipment:

   - A positive-pressure oxygen delivery system suitable for the patient being treated must be immediately available.
   - Documentation of compliance with manufacturers' recommended maintenance of monitors, anesthesia delivery systems, and other anesthesia-related equipment should be maintained. A pre-procedural check of equipment for each administration of sedation must be performed.
   - When inhalation equipment is used, it must have a fail-safe system that is appropriately checked and calibrated. The equipment must also have either (1) a functioning device that prohibits the delivery of less than 30% oxygen or (2) an appropriately calibrated and functioning in-line oxygen analyzer with audible alarm.
   - An appropriate scavenging system must be available if gases other than oxygen or air are used.

4. **Monitoring and Documentation**

   Monitoring: A dentist, or at the dentist's direction, an appropriately trained individual, must remain in the operatory during active dental treatment to monitor the patient continuously until the patient meets the criteria for discharge to the recovery area. The appropriately trained individual must be familiar with monitoring techniques and equipment. Monitoring must include:

   - *Consciousness:* Level of sedation (e.g., responsiveness to verbal commands) must be continually assessed.
   - *Oxygenation:* Oxygen saturation by pulse oximetry may be clinically useful and should be considered.
   - *Ventilation:*
     - The dentist and/or appropriately trained individual must observe chest excursions.
     - The dentist and/or appropriately trained individual must verify respirations.
   - *Circulation:* Blood pressure and heart rate should be evaluated pre-operatively, postoperatively and intraoperatively as necessary (unless the patient is unable to tolerate such monitoring).

   Documentation: An appropriate sedative record must be maintained, including the names of all drugs administered, time administered and route of administration, including local anesthetics, dosages, and monitored physiological parameters.

5. Recovery and Discharge

- Oxygen and suction equipment must be immediately available if a separate recovery area is utilized.
- The qualified dentist or appropriately trained clinical staff must monitor the patient during recovery until the patient is ready for discharge by the dentist.
- The qualified dentist must determine and document that level of consciousness, oxygenation, ventilation and circulation are satisfactory prior to discharge.
- Postoperative verbal and written instructions must be given to the patient, parent, escort, legal guardian or care giver.

6. Emergency Management

- If a patient enters a deeper level of sedation than the dentist is qualified to provide, the dentist must stop the dental procedure until the patient returns is returned to the intended level of sedation.
- The qualified dentist is responsible for the sedative management, adequacy of the facility and staff, diagnosis and treatment of emergencies related to the administration of minimal sedation and providing the equipment and protocols for patient rescue.

B. Moderate Sedation

1. Patient History and Evaluation

Patients considered for moderate sedation must undergo an evaluation prior to the administration of any sedative. This should consist of at least a review at an appropriate time of their medical history and medication use and NPO (nothing by mouth) status. In addition, patients with significant medical considerations (e.g., ASA III, IV)[2] should also require consultation with their primary care physician or consulting medical specialist. Assessment of Body Mass Index (BMI)4 should be considered part of a pre-procedural workup. Patients with elevated BMI may be at increased risk for airway associated morbidity, particularly if in association with other factors such as obstructive sleep apnea.

2. Preoperative Evaluation and Preparation

- The patient, parent, legal guardian or caregiver must be advised regarding the procedure associated with the delivery of any sedative agents and informed consent for the proposed sedation must be obtained.
- Determination of adequate oxygen supply and equipment necessary to deliver oxygen under positive pressure must be completed.
- An appropriate focused physical evaluation must be performed.
- Baseline vital signs including body weight, height, blood pressure, pulse rate, respiration rate, and blood oxygen saturation by pulse oximetry must be obtained unless precluded by the nature of the patient,

procedure or equipment. Body temperature should be measured when clinically indicated.

- Preoperative verbal or written instructions must be given to the patient, parent, escort, legal guardian or care giver, including preoperative fasting instructions based on the ASA Summary of Fasting and Pharmacologic Recommendations.

3. **Personnel and Equipment Requirements**

   Personnel: At least one additional person trained in Basic Life Support for Healthcare Providers must be present in addition to the dentist.

   Equipment:

   - A positive-pressure oxygen delivery system suitable for the patient being treated must be immediately available.

   - Documentation of compliance with manufacturers' recommended maintenance of monitors, anesthesia delivery systems, and other anesthesia-related equipment should be maintained. A pre-procedural check of equipment for each administration of sedation must be performed.

   - When inhalation equipment is used, it must have a fail-safe system that is appropriately checked and calibrated. The equipment must also have either (1) a functioning device that prohibits the delivery of less than 30% oxygen or (2) an appropriately calibrated and functioning in-line oxygen analyzer with audible alarm.

   - The equipment necessary for monitoring end-tidal CO_2 and auscultation of breath sounds must be immediately available.

   - An appropriate scavenging system must be available if gases other than oxygen or air are used.

   - The equipment necessary to establish intravascular or intraosseous access should be available until the patient meets discharge criteria.

4. **Monitoring and Documentation**

   Monitoring: A qualified dentist administering moderate sedation must remain in the operatory room to monitor the patient continuously until the patient meets the criteria for recovery. When active treatment concludes and the patient recovers to a minimally sedated level a qualified auxiliary may be directed by the dentist to remain with the patient and continue to monitor them as explained in the guidelines until they are discharged from the facility. The dentist must not leave the facility until the patient meets the criteria for discharge and is discharged from the facility. Monitoring must include:

   - *Consciousness:* Level of sedation (e.g., responsiveness to verbal command) must be continually assessed.

   - *Oxygenation:* Oxygen saturation must be evaluated by pulse oximetry continuously.

- *Ventilation:*
  - The dentist must observe chest excursions continually.
  - The dentist must monitor ventilation and/or breathing by monitoring end-tidal CO_2 unless precluded or invalidated by the nature of the patient, procedure or equipment. In addition, ventilation should be monitored by continual observation of qualitative signs, including auscultation of breath sounds with a precordial or pretracheal stethoscope.
- *Circulation:*
  - The dentist must continually evaluate blood pressure and heart rate unless invalidated by the nature of the patient, procedure or equipment and this is noted in the time-oriented anesthesia record.
  - Continuous ECG monitoring of patients with significant cardiovascular disease should be considered.

Documentation:

- Appropriate time-oriented anesthetic record must be maintained, including the names of all drugs, dosages and their administration times, including local anesthetics, dosages and monitored physiological parameters.
- Pulse oximetry, heart rate, respiratory rate, blood pressure and level of consciousness must be recorded continually.

5. **Recovery and Discharge**

- Oxygen and suction equipment must be immediately available if a separate recovery area is utilized.
- The qualified dentist or appropriately trained clinical staff must continually monitor the patient's blood pressure, heart rate, oxygenation and level of consciousness.
- The qualified dentist must determine and document that level of consciousness; oxygenation, ventilation and circulation are satisfactory for discharge.
- Postoperative verbal and written instructions must be given to the patient, parent, escort, legal guardian or caregiver.
- If a pharmacological reversal agent is administered before discharge criteria have been met, the patient must be monitored for a longer period than usual before discharge, since re-sedation may occur once the effects of the reversal agent have waned.

6. **Emergency Management**

- If a patient enters a deeper level of sedation than the dentist is qualified to provide, the dentist must stop the dental procedure until the patient is returned to the intended level of sedation.
- The qualified dentist is responsible for the sedative management, adequacy of the facility and staff, diagnosis and treatment of emergencies related to the administration of moderate sedation and providing the equipment, drugs and protocol for patient rescue.

C. Deep Sedation or General Anesthesia

1. Patient History and Evaluation

Patients considered for deep sedation or general anesthesia must undergo an evaluation prior to the administration of any sedative. This must consist of at least a review of their medical history and medication use and NPO (nothing by mouth) status. In addition, patients with significant medical considerations (e.g., ASA III, IV)[2] should also require consultation with their primary care physician or consulting medical specialist. Assessment of Body Mass Index (BMI)[4] should be considered part of a pre-procedural workup. Patients with elevated BMI may be at increased risk for airway associated morbidity, particularly if in association with other factors such as obstructive sleep apnea.

2. Preoperative Evaluation and Preparation

- The patient, parent, legal guardian or caregiver must be advised regarding the procedure associated with the delivery of any sedative or anesthetic agents and informed consent for the proposed sedation/anesthesia must be obtained.

- Determination of adequate oxygen supply and equipment necessary to deliver oxygen under positive pressure must be completed.

- A focused physical evaluation must be performed as deemed appropriate.

- Baseline vital signs including body weight, height, blood pressure, pulse rate, respiration rate, and blood oxygen saturation by pulse oximetry must be obtained unless invalidated by the patient, procedure or equipment. In addition, body temperature should be measured when clinically appropriate.

- Preoperative verbal and written instructions must be given to the patient, parent, escort, legal guardian or care giver, including pre-operative fasting instructions based on the ASA Summary of Fasting and Pharmacologic Recommendations.

- An intravenous line, which is secured throughout the procedure, must be established except as provided in part IV. C.6., Special Needs Patients, of the ADA Guidelines.[1]

3. Personnel and Equipment Requirements

Personnel: A minimum of three (3) individuals must be present:

- A dentist qualified in accordance with part IV. C. of the ADA Guidelines[1] to administer the deep sedation or general anesthesia.

- Two additional individuals who have current certification of successfully completing a Basic Life Support (BLS) Course for the Healthcare Provider.

- When the same individual administering the deep sedation or general anesthesia is performing the dental procedure, one of the additional appropriately trained team members must be designated for patient monitoring.

Equipment:

- A positive-pressure oxygen delivery system suitable for the patient being treated must be immediately available.

- Documentation of compliance with manufacturers' recommended maintenance of monitors, anesthesia delivery systems, and other anesthesia-related equipment should be maintained. A pre-procedural check of equipment for each administration must be performed.

- When inhalation equipment is used, it must have a fail-safe system that is appropriately checked and calibrated. The equipment must also have either (1) a functioning device that prohibits the delivery of less than 30% oxygen or (2) an appropriately calibrated and functioning in-line oxygen analyzer with audible alarm.

- An appropriate scavenging system must be available if gases other than oxygen or air are used.

- The equipment necessary to establish intravenous access must be available.

- Equipment and drugs necessary to provide advanced airway management, and advanced cardiac life support must be immediately available.

- The equipment necessary for monitoring end-tidal CO_2 and auscultation of breath sounds must be immediately available.

- Resuscitation medications and an appropriate defibrillator must be immediately available.

4. **Monitoring and Documentation**

   Monitoring: A qualified dentist administering deep sedation or general anesthesia must remain in the operatory room to monitor the patient continuously until the patient meets the criteria for recovery. The dentist must not leave the facility until the patient meets the criteria for discharge and is discharged from the facility. Monitoring must include:

   - *Oxygenation:* Oxygenation saturation must be evaluated continuously by pulse oximetry.

   - *Ventilation:*

     - Intubated patient: End-tidal CO_2 must be continuously monitored and evaluated.

     - Non-intubated patient: End-tidal CO_2 must be continually monitored and evaluated unless precluded or invalidated by the nature of the patient, procedure, or equipment. In addition, ventilation should be monitored and evaluated by continual observation of qualitative signs, including auscultation of breath sounds with a precordial or pretracheal stethoscope.

     - Respiration rate must be continually monitored and evaluated.

   - *Circulation:*

     - The dentist must continuously evaluate heart rate and rhythm via ECG throughout the procedure, as well as pulse rate via pulse oximetry.

     - The dentist must continually evaluate blood pressure.

- *Temperature:*
  - A device capable of measuring body temperature must be readily available during the administration of deep sedation or general anesthesia.
  - The equipment to continuously monitor body temperature should be available and must be performed whenever triggering agents associated with malignant hyperthermia are administered.
- *Documentation:*
  - Appropriate time-oriented anesthetic record must be maintained, including the names of all drugs, dosages and their administration times, including local anesthetics and monitored physiological parameters.
  - Pulse oximetry and end-tidal CO_2 measurements (if taken), heart rate, respiratory rate and blood pressure must be recorded continually.

5. **Recovery and Discharge**
   - Oxygen and suction equipment must be immediately available if a separate recovery area is utilized.
   - The dentist or clinical staff must continually monitor the patient's blood pressure, heart rate, oxygenation and level of consciousness.
   - The dentist must determine and document that level of consciousness; oxygenation, ventilation and circulation are satisfactory for discharge.
   - Postoperative verbal and written instructions must be given to the patient, and parent, escort, guardian or care giver.

6. **Special Needs Patients**

   Because many dental patients undergoing deep sedation or general anesthesia are mentally and/or physically challenged, it is not always possible to have a comprehensive physical examination or appropriate laboratory tests prior to administering care. When these situations occur, the dentist responsible for administering the deep sedation or general anesthesia should document the reasons preventing the recommended preoperative management.

   In selected circumstances, deep sedation or general anesthesia may be utilized without establishing an indwelling intravenous line. These selected circumstances may include very brief procedures or periods of time, which, for example, may occur in some patients; or the establishment of intravenous access after deep sedation or general anesthesia has been induced because of poor patient cooperation.

7. **Emergency Management**

   The qualified dentist is responsible for sedative/anesthetic management, adequacy of the facility and staff, diagnosis and treatment of emergencies related to the administration of deep sedation or general anesthesia and providing the equipment, drugs and protocols for patient rescue.

1. American Dental Association. Guidelines for the Use of Sedation and General Anesthesia by Dentists. Adopted by the ADA House of Delegates, October 2016.

2. American Society of Anesthesiologists. ASA Physical Status Classification System (Updated by ASA House of Delegates October 15, 2014). Available at *https://www.asahq.org/resources/clinical-information/asa-physical-status-classification-system*. Accessed August 3, 2018.

* Additional Endnotes

Excerpted from Continuum of Depth of Sedation: Definition of General Anesthesia and Levels of Sedation/Analgesia, 2014, of the American Society of Anesthesiologists. A copy of the full text can be obtained from ASA, 1061 American Lane Schaumburg, IL 60173-4973 or online at *http://www.asahq.org/quality-and-practice-management/standards-guidelines-and-related-resources/continuum-of-depth-of-sedation-definition-of-general-anesthesia-and-levels-of-sedation-analgesia*.

Excerpted from American Society of Anesthesiologists: Practice Guidelines for preoperative fasting and the use of pharmacologic agents to reduce the risk of pulmonary aspiration: application to healthy patients undergoing elective procedures. Anesthesiology, 2011. A copy of the full text can be obtained from ASA, 1061 American Lane Schaumburg, IL 60173-4973 or online at *http://anesthesiology.pubs.asahq.org/article.aspx?articleid=2596245&_ga=2.112974276.1177752640.1534960138-743492268.1533328211*.

Standardized BMI category definitions can be obtained from the Centers for Disease Control and Prevention or the American Society of Anesthesiologists.

Section 4:

Guidance in Specific Populations: Pregnancy, Elderly and Substance Abuse

Prepared by Kathleen Ziegler, PharmD

Pregnancy and Breastfeeding

Oral health care, including having dental radiographs taken and being given local anesthesia, is safe at any point during pregnancy. Further, the American Dental Association and the American Congress (formerly "College") of Obstetricians and Gynecologists (ACOG) agree that emergency treatments, such as extractions, root canals or restorations can be safely performed during pregnancy and that delaying treatment may result in more complex problems.

When treating pregnant patients, it might be helpful to reach out to the obstetrician to develop a working relationship should consultation be needed later. Questions you might ask include:

- When is the expected delivery date?
- Is this a high-risk pregnancy? If so, are there any special concerns or contraindications?

Questions about the local anesthetics or antibiotics used in dentistry are common when treating this patient population. According to a 2012 JADA article by Donaldson and Goodchild (see Suggested Reading List), options considered safe for use in these situations include certain local anesthetics (with or without epinephrine), most antibiotics, and some pain relievers (see Table 1).

Table 1. Key Medication Considerations During Pregnancy and Breastfeeding**			
Medication Type	**FDA Pregnancy Risk Category**	**Safe During Pregnancy?**	**Safe During Breastfeeding?**
Analgesics and Anti-inflammatories*			
Acetaminophen	B	Yes	Yes
Aspirin	C/D	Avoid	Avoid
Codeine	C	Use with caution	No[†]
Glucocorticoids (e.g., prednisone)	C	Avoid[‡]	Yes
Hydrocodone	C	Use with caution	Use with caution
Ibuprofen[§]	C/D	Avoid use in third trimester	Yes
Oxycodone	B	Use with caution	Use with caution
Antibiotics[¶#]			
Amoxicillin	B	Yes	Yes
Azithromycin	B	Yes	Yes
Cephalexin	B	Yes	Yes
Chlorhexidine (topical)	B	Yes	Yes
Clarithromycin	C	Use with caution	Use with caution
Clindamycin	B	Yes	Yes
Clotrimazole (topical)	B	Yes	Yes
Doxycycline	D	Avoid	Avoid
Erythromycin	B	Yes	Use with caution
Fluconazole	C/D	Yes (single-dose regimens)	Yes
Metronidazole	B	Yes	Avoid; may give breast milk an unpleasant taste
Nystatin	C	Yes	Yes
Penicillin	B	Yes	Yes
Terconazole (topical)	B	Yes	Yes
Tetracycline	D	Avoid	Avoid
Local Anesthetics			
Articaine	C	Use with caution	Use with caution
Bupivacaine	C	Use with caution	Yes
Lidocaine (+/- epinephrine)	B	Yes	Yes
Mepivacaine (+/- levonordefrin)	C	Use with caution	Yes
Prilocaine	B	Yes	Yes

Table 1. Key Medication Considerations During Pregnancy and Breastfeeding**			
Medication Type	FDA Pregnancy Risk Category	Safe During Pregnancy?	Safe During Breastfeeding?
Benzocaine (topical)	C	Use with caution	Use with caution
Dyclonine (topical)	C	Yes	Yes
Lidocaine (topical)	B	Yes	Yes
Tetracaine (topical)	C	Use with caution	Use with caution
Sedatives			
Benzodiazepines	D/X	Avoid	Avoid
Zaleplon	C	Use with caution	Use with caution
Zolpidem	C	Use with caution	Yes
Emergency Medications			
Albuterol	C	Steroid and β2-agonist inhalers are safe	Yes
Diphenhydramine	B	Yes	Avoid
Epinephrine	C	Use with caution	Yes
Flumazenil	C	Use with caution	Use with caution
Naloxone	C	Use with caution	Use with caution
Nitroglycerin	C	Use with caution	Use with caution

* In the case of combination products (such as oxycodone with acetaminophen), the safety with respect to either pregnancy or breastfeeding is dependent on the higher-risk moiety. In the example of oxycodone with acetaminophen, the combination of these two drugs should be used with caution, because the oxycodone moiety carries a higher risk than the acetaminophen moiety.

† In April 2017, the U.S. Food and Drug Administration issued a warning that recommends against use of codeine and tramadol in children younger than 12 years, also extending the warning against use to breastfeeding women because of possible harm to infants.

‡ Oral steroids should not be withheld from patients with acute severe asthma.

§ Ibuprofen is representative of all nonsteroidal anti-inflammatory drugs. In breastfeeding patients, avoid cyclooxygenase selective inhibitors such as celecoxib, as few data regarding their safe use in this population are available, and avoid doses of aspirin higher than 100 milligrams because of risk of platelet dysfunction and Reye syndrome.

¶ Antibiotic use during pregnancy: The patient should receive the full adult dose and for the usual length of treatment. Serious infections should be treated aggressively. Penicillins and cephalosporins are considered safe. Use higher-dose regimens (such as cephalexin 500 mg three times per day rather than 250 mg three times per day), as they are cleared from the system more quickly because of the increase in glomerular filtration rate in pregnancy.

Antibiotic use during breastfeeding: These agents may cause altered bowel flora and, thus, diarrhea in the baby. If the infant develops a fever, the clinician should take into account maternal antibiotic treatment.

**Adapted with permission from Donaldson M, Goodchild JH. Pregnancy, breast-feeding and drugs used in dentistry. J Am Dent Assoc 2012;143(8):858-71.

1 | Medication Use in Pregnancy

Providing needed dental treatment, managing oral infection, and controlling pain are essential functions of dentists for helping patients maintain overall health during pregnancy. For a pregnant patient requiring dental care, the agents prescribed should be especially evaluated for potential risks to the mother and/or fetus. The decision to administer a specific drug requires that the benefits outweigh the potential risks of therapy.

Historically, manufacturers have relied on an alphabetical system to communicate the safety of medications for use with pregnant patients (Table 2). In 2015, the US. Food & Drug Administration began phasing out that system for prescription drugs, replacing it with a narrative section in the package insert that discusses the benefits and risks of using a particular medication with this population. The new system will be phased-in, with a full compliance date of 2020. After 2020, the alphabetical system will continue to be used for over-the-counter medications.

2 | Medication Use During Breastfeeding

Drugs that negatively impact pregnancy are not necessarily unsafe during breastfeeding. According to the American Academy of Pediatrics Committee Report on Drugs, many drugs "should not affect the milk supply or breast-feeding infant." (see Suggested Reading List).

One option women have when faced with taking medications is to pump and save milk prior to the dental appointment; then, pump and discard the milk produced after use of medication. Donaldson and Goodchild suggest that this approach is especially useful when drugs with short half-lives are used. They report that it takes approximately four half-lives to eliminate more than 90 percent of most medications. (see Suggested Reading List).

Questions also often arise about medication use by patients who are lactating. Most medication product inserts have information related to use during lactation. The National Library of Medicine also provides a searchable database (LactMed) on this topic.

3 | Analgesia and Anesthesia Safety Issues

Many analgesics are available over-the-counter, providing easy access and perhaps even the implication that these medications are safe when taken during pregnancy or breastfeeding. According to Donaldson and Goodchild, however, some of these medications can be harmful to the fetus, mother or infant if used during these periods (see Suggested Reading List). For example, they report that ibuprofen has been known to have detrimental effects when taken during pregnancy such as problems in fetal implantation, childbirth and maternal pulmonary hypertension. Aspirin has been linked to development of fetal organs outside the abdominal wall when taken during pregnancy, according to the authors.

Aspirin also presents risks when used during breastfeeding, including bleeding and Reye Syndrome, and thus, should be avoided. According the American Academy of Pediatrics Committee on Drugs, acetaminophen is a better option for pain relief for women who are breast feeding.

Nitrous oxide is classified as a pregnancy risk group Category C medication, meaning that there is a risk of fetal harm if administered during pregnancy. It is recommended that pregnant women, both patients and staff, avoid exposure to nitrous oxide.

Table 2. Drug Category and Evidence of Pregnancy Risk

Category A	Controlled studies show no risk
Category B	No evidence of risk in humans • Adequate well-controlled studies in pregnant women have not shown increased risk of fetal abnormalities despite adverse findings in animals. OR • In the absence of human studies, animal studies showed no fetal risk. The chance of fetal harm is remote but remains a possibility.
Category C	Risk cannot be ruled out • Adequate well-controlled human studies are lacking, and animal studies have shown a risk to the fetus or are lacking as well. There is a chance of fetal harm if administered during pregnancy, but the potential benefits may outweigh the potential risk.
Category D	Positive evidence of risk • Studies in humans, or investigational or post-marketing data, have demonstrated fetal risk. Nevertheless, potential benefits from use of this drug may outweigh the potential risk. For example, the drug may be acceptable if needed in a life-threatening situation or serious disease for which safer drugs cannot be used or are ineffective.
Category X	Contraindicated in pregnancy • Studies in animals or humans, investigational or postmarketing reports, have demonstrated positive evidence of fetal abnormalities or risk that clearly outweighs any possible benefit to the patient.

Suggested Reading

- Donaldson M, Goodchild JH. Pregnancy, breast-feeding and drugs used in dentistry. J Am Dent Assoc 2012;143(8):858-71.
- American Association of Pediatrics Committee on Drugs. The Transfer of Drugs and Other Chemicals into Human Milk. Pediatrics 2001;108(3):776-789.
- ACOG Committee Opinion No. 569: oral health care during pregnancy and through the lifespan. Obstet Gynecol 2013;122(2 Pt 1):417-22.
- Steinberg BJ, Hilton IV, Iida H, Samelson R. Oral health and dental care during pregnancy. Dent Clin North Am 2013;57(2):195-210.
- Hagai A, Diav-Citrin O, Shechtman S, Ornoy A. Pregnancy outcome after in utero exposure to local anesthetics as part of dental treatment: A prospective comparative cohort study. J Am Dent Assoc 2015;146(8):572-80.
- Mendia J, Cuddy MA, Moore PA. Drug therapy for the pregnant dental patient. Compend Contin Educ Dent 2012;33(8):568-70, 72, 74-6 passim; quiz 79, 96.

The Elderly and Medication Considerations

According to data from National Health and Nutrition Examination Survey (NHANES), 39% of people aged 65 years and older reported using 5 or more prescription drugs ("polypharmacy") in the prior 30 days during the years 2011 through 2012. Ninety percent of people 65 years of age and older reported using any prescription drug in the prior 30 days. The high prevalence of polypharmacy among older adults may lead to inappropriate drug use, medication errors, drug interactions or adverse drug reactions. According to Ouanounou and Haasthe, the average older adult takes 4 or 5 prescription drugs; in addition, these individuals may also be taking 2 or 3 over-the-counter (OTC) medications (see Suggested Reading List). A review of older dental patients' medical history and current medications, both prescription and OTC medications/supplements, should be done regularly.

1 | Medication Considerations

Drugs most commonly prescribed in elderly patients include "statin" drugs for hypercholesterolemia; antihypertensive agents; analgesics; drugs for endocrine dysfunction, including thyroid and diabetes medications; antiplatelet agents or anticoagulants; drugs for respiratory conditions (e.g., albuterol); antidepressants; antibiotics; and drugs for gastroesophageal reflux disease and acid reflux. The most frequently taken OTC medications by older adults include analgesics, laxatives, vitamins, and minerals.

Older adults frequently show an exaggerated response to central nervous system drugs, partly resulting from an age-related decline in central nervous system function and partly resulting from increased sensitivity to certain benzodiazepines, general anesthetics, and opioids. The American Geriatrics Society has published a 2015 update to the Beers Criteria for potentially inappropriate medication use in older adults have been found to be associated with poor health outcomes, including confusion, falls, and mortality (see Suggested Reading List). One change of note to the 2015 Beers Criteria includes the addition of opioids to the category of central nervous system medications that should be avoided in individuals with a history of falls or fractures. Check out the Latest Prescribing Recommendations in the Elderly before prescribing or administering medications to your senior patients, which can be found here:

www.guideline.gov/summaries/summary/49933/american-geriatrics-society-2015-updated-beers-criteria-for-potentially-inappropriate-medication-use-in-older-adults

2 | Oral Health and General Dental Considerations

Xerostomia affects 30% of patients older than 65 years and up to 40% of patients older than 80 years; this is primarily an adverse effect of medication(s), although it can also result from comorbid conditions such as diabetes, Alzheimer's disease, or Parkinson's disease.

Xerostomia, while common among older patients, is more likely to result from medication use. Dry mouth can lead to mucositis, caries, cracked lips, and fissured tongue. Stein and Alaboe suggest that individuals with dry mouth consider drinking or at least sipping regular water throughout the day and limiting alcoholic beverages and beverages high in sugar or caffeine, such as juices, sodas, teas or coffee (especially sweetened) (see Suggested Reading List).

Because cardiovascular disease is common among older individuals, it has been suggested by Ouanounou and Haas that the dose of epinephrine contained in anesthetics should be limited to a maximum of 0.04 mg (see Suggested Reading List). The authors recommend that even without a history of overt cardiovascular disease, the use of epinephrine in older adult patients should be minimized because of the expected effect of aging on the heart. They recommend monitoring blood pressure and heart rate when considering multiple administrations of epinephrine-containing local anesthetic in the older adult population.

Suggested Reading

- Ouanounou A, Haas DA. Pharmacotherapy for the elderly dental patient. J Can Dent Assoc 2015;80:f18.

- Fitzgerald J, Epstein JB, Donaldson M, et al. Outpatient medication use and implications for dental care: guidance for contemporary dental practice. J Can Dent Assoc 2015;81:f10.

- Bowie MW, Slattum PW. Pharmacodynamics in older adults: a review. Am J Geriatr Pharmacother 2007;5(3):263-303.

- American Geriatrics Society 2015 Updated Beers Criteria for Potentially Inappropriate Medication Use in Older Adults. J Am Geriatr Soc 2015.

- Razak PA, Richard KM, Thankachan RP, et al. Geriatric oral health: a review article. J Int Oral Health 2014;6(6):110-6.

- Preston AJ. Dental management of the elderly patient. Dent Update 2012;39(2):141-3.

- Stein P, Aalboe J. Dental care in the frail older adult: special considerations and recommendations. J Calif Dent Assoc 2015;43(7):363-8.45.

Substance Abuse Disorder

Box 1. Pain Management in Substance Abuse Disorders

Clinical Considerations Prior to Administering or Prescribing to Patients with a History of Substance Abuse Disorders*

Q: Is the medication in the class of medications or substances that was/is the patient's preferred substance of abuse?
A: If yes, do you absolutely need to administer or prescribe this medication? (Addiction IS NOT a contraindication to prescribe the medication if the benefits outweigh the risks.)

Q: Is the patient in a treatment program for drug or alcohol addiction or under a treatment center/prescriber contract for pain or anxiety management?
A: If yes, dental practitioners optimally should consult with the treatment center or practitioner enforcing the contract to discuss preferred treatment options.

Q: Will the medication being administered result in a positive drug screen that potentially could compromise treatment contracts?
A: If yes, dental practitioners and patients should discuss this issue with personnel responsible for the treatment contract before the procedure when possible.

[Nonsteroidal anti-inflammatory drugs] remain the first-line oral agents of choice for the management of acute pain in dental procedures unless otherwise contraindicated.

For patients with a history of alcohol, benzodiazepine, or barbiturate addition, controlled substances such as benzodiazepines or barbiturates are not recommended for light sedation or anxiolysis due to the potential for stimulating similar pathways in the brain that promote craving.

Alternative agents, such as antihistamines (diphenhydramine or hydroxyzine), may be considered if light sedation is required. Anecdotally, patients in recovery from alcohol or benzodiazepine addiction have reported a significant increase in cravings after receiving nitrous oxide inhalation for light sedation or anxiolysis.

* Adapted from O'Neil M, ed. The ADA Practical Guide to Substance Use Disorders and Safe Prescribing. Hoboken, NJ: John Wiley & Sons, Inc.; 2015.

Suggested Reading

· O'Neil M, ed. The ADA Practical Guide to Substance Use Disorders and Safe Prescribing. Hoboken, NJ: John Wiley & Sons, Inc.; 2015.

Useful Tables

1. Adverse Drug Reactions (Oral)
2. Drug-Drug Interactions
3. Generic – Brand List

Prepared by Jay Elkareh, PharmD, PhD, ADA Science Institute

Table 1. Adverse Drug Reactions (Oral)

Oral Manifestations of Drug Reactions	Most Common Prescribed Drugs in 2017									
	Alprazolam	Amlodipine	Amoxicillin	Atorvastatin	Azithromycin	Furosemide	Gabapentin	Hydrochloro-thiazide	Hydrocodone/APAP	Ibuprofen
Angioedema										
Bleeding				●						●
Candidiasis			●		●		●			
Canker Sores		●					●			
Cough				●	●		●		●	
Dental Caries										
Dry Mouth (Xerostomia)	●			●		●	●			
Facial Paralysis				●						
Gingival Enlargement										
Gingival Inflammation (Gingivitis)							●			
Herpes Simplex							●			
Hemostasis Impairment							●			
Larynx Inflammation (Laryngitis)							●			
Lips Inflammation (Cheilitis)				●			●			
Mouth Inflammation (Stomatitis)			●	●	●		●			
Orofacial Pain	●					●				
Osteonecrosis	●			●			●			
Swallowing Difficulty (Dysphagia)	●									
Tardive Dyskinesia										
Taste Alteration (Dysgeusia)	●	●		●	●		●			
Taste Loss (Ageusia)				●	●		●			
Throat Soarness (Pharyngitis)							●			
Tongue Disorder			●	●			●			
Tongue Inflammation (Glossitis)							●			
Tooth Discoloration			●				●			

Suggested Reading: Ciancio S, ed. ADA/PDR Guide to dental therapeutics. Fifth ed. Chicago: American Dental Association, 2009 Chap 24. Oral manifestations of systemic agents.

Table 1. Adverse Drug Reactions (Oral)

Most Common Prescribed Drugs in 2017

Oral Manifestations of Drug Reactions	Levothyroxine	Lisinopril	Losartan	Metformin	Metoprolol	Omeprazole	Ondansetron	Prednisone	Sertraline	Zolpidem
Angioedema		✓	✓							✓
Bleeding										
Candidiasis										
Canker Sores										
Cough		✓	✓			✓			✓	✓
Dental Caries					✓				✓	✓
Dry Mouth (Xerostomia)		✓	✓			✓	✓		✓	
Facial Paralysis										
Gingival Enlargement										
Gingival Inflammation (Gingivitis)										
Herpes Simplex								✓		
Hemostasis Impairment										
Larynx Inflammation (Laryngitis)		✓								
Lips Inflammation (Cheilitis)		✓	✓							
Mouth Inflammation (Stomatitis)										
Orofacial Pain		✓	✓			✓			✓	✓
Osteonecrosis		✓								
Swallowing Difficulty (Dysphagia)										
Tardive Dyskinesia										
Taste Alteration (Dysgeusia)		✓	✓	✓	✓	✓			✓	✓
Taste Loss (Ageusia)		✓	✓							
Throat Soarness (Pharyngitis)		✓			✓	✓			✓	✓
Tongue Disorder						✓			✓	
Tongue Inflammation (Glossitis)									✓	
Tooth Discoloration										

Table 2. Drug-Drug Interactions

Most common prescribed drugs in dental medicine	Alprazolam	Amlodipine	Amoxicillin	Atorvastatin	Azithromycin	Furosemide	Gabapentin	Hydrochloro-thiazide	Hydrocodone/APAP	Ibuprofen
Analgesics										
Acetaminophen							X			
Aspirin			X			X		X		XX
Celecoxib						X		X	X	X
Ibuprofen						X		X		
Naproxen						X		X		XX
Codeine	X								X	
Hydrocodone	XX							XX		
Hydromorphone	X								X	
Oxycodone	X								X	
Tramadol	X								XX	
Anesthetics										
Articaine										
Bupivacaine										
Lidocaine									X	
Mepivacaine										
Prilocaine										
Phentolamine		X								X
Antibiotics										
Amoxicillin					X			X		
Azithromycin			X	X						
Clindamycin										
Doxycycline			XX							
Erythromycin	XX	X	X	XX	X					
Metronidazole	XX	X		X						X
Penicillin VK						X	X	X		
Antifungals										
Clotrimazole				X	X					
Fluconazole	X	X		X	X					X
Nystatin										
Voriconazole	X	X		X	X				XX	X
Antivirals										
Acyclovir			X					X		X
ValAcyclovir										
Anxiolytics										
Diazepam	X								XX	
Triazolam	X								XX	
Corticosteroids										
Dexamethasone	X	X		X		X		X	XX	X

Legend: **X** - Monitor   **XX** - Avoid   **XXX** - Contraindicated

158

Table 2. Drug-Drug Interactions

Most common prescribed drugs in dental medicine	Levothyroxine	Lisinopril	Losartan	Metformin	Metoprolol	Omeprazole	Ondansetron	Prednisone	Sertraline	Zolpidem
Analgesics										
Acetaminophen										
Aspirin		XX	X		X			X	X	
Celecoxib		XX	X		X			X	X	
Ibuprofen		XX	X		X			X	X	
Naproxen		XX	X		X			X	X	
Codeine									X	
Hydrocodone									X	
Hydromorphone									XX	
Oxycodone									X	XX
Tramadol									X	
Anesthetics										
Articaine										
Bupivacaine										
Lidocaine						X				
Mepivacaine										
Prilocaine										
Phentolamine		X			X					
Antibiotics										
Amoxicillin										
Azithromycin							XX			
Clindamycin										
Doxycycline										
Erythromycin							XX	XX		X
Metronidazole			X					X		X
Penicillin VK										
Antifungals										
Clotrimazole								X		
Fluconazole			X			X	XX	X		X
Nystatin										
Voriconazole			X			X	XX	X		X
Antivirals										
Acyclovir										
ValAcyclovir										
Anxiolytics										
Diazepam					X	X		X		X
Triazolam						X		X		X
Corticosteroids										
Dexamethasone				X		X	X	X		X

Legend: **X** - Monitor **XX** - Avoid **XXX** - Contraindicated

Table 2. Drug-Drug Interactions

Most common prescribed drugs in dental medicine	Most Common Prescribed Drugs in 2017									
	Alprazolam	Amlodipine	Amoxicillin	Atorvastatin	Azithromycin	Furosemide	Gabapentin	Hydrochloro-thiazide	Hydrocodone/APAP	Ibuprofen
Emergency Drugs										
Albuterol	X					X		X	X	X
Atropine										
Diphenhydramine	X								X	
Ephedrine	X					X		X	X	X
Ephinephrine	X				X	X		X	X	
Flumazenil										
Hydrocortisone	X	X		X		X		X		X
Lorazepam	X								X	
Naloxone									X	
Nitroglycerin										
Fluoride										
Muscle Relaxants										
Baclofen	X									
Carisoprodol	X								X	
Cyclobenzaprine	X								X	
Metaxalone	X								X	
Orphenadrine	X								X	
Tizanidine		X				X		X		
Salivary Management										
Cevimeline										
Pilocarpine										
Glycopyrrolate										
Tobacco Cessation										
Nicotine										
Bupropion									X	
Varenicline										

Legend: **X** - Monitor   **XX** - Avoid   **XXX** - Contraindicated

Table 2. Drug-Drug Interactions

Most common prescribed drugs in dental medicine	Levothyroxine	Lisinopril	Losartan	Metformin	Metoprolol	Omeprazole	Ondansetron	Prednisone	Sertraline	Zolpidem
Emergency Drugs										
Albuterol					X					
Atropine										
Diphenydramine					X					
Ephedrine					X					
Ephinephrine					X					
Flumazenil										
Hydrocortisone				X				X		X
Lorazepam						X				
Naloxone										
Nitroglycerin										
Fluoride										
Muscle Relaxants										
Baclofen										
Carisoprodol										
Cyclobenzaprine									XX	
Metaxalone										
Orphenadrine										
Tizanidine		X	X		X	X				
Salivary Management										
Cevimeline					X			X		
Pilocarpine					X					
Glycopyrrolate				X						
Tobacco Cessation										
Nicotine										
Bupropion				X					X	
Varenicline										

Legend: **X** - Monitor   **XX** - Avoid   **XXX** - Contraindicated

Table 3a. Most Common Prescribed Drugs in Dental Medicine

Generic	Brand Names
Analgesics	
Acetaminophen (APAP)	Tylenol
Aspirin (ASA)	Aspirin
Celecoxib	Celebrex
Ibuprofen	Motrin
Naproxen	Aleve, Anaprox, Naprosyn
Codeine	Codeine
Codeine/APAP	Tylenol #2, Tylenol #3, Tylenol #4
Hydromorphone	Dilaudid
Hydrocodone	Zohydro (ER)
Hydrocodone/APAP	Lortab, Norco, Vicodin
Hydrocodone/Ibuprofen	Vicoprofen
Hydromorphone	Dilaudid
Oxycodone	Roxicodone, Oxycontin (ER)
Oxycodone/APAP	Percocet, Roxicet
Oxycodone/Ibuprofen	Combunox
Tramadol	Ultram
Tramadol/APAP	Ultracet
Anesthetics	
Articaine	Septocaine, Ultracaine, Articadent, Zorcaine
Bupivacaine	Marcaine, Vivacaine, Sensorcaine
Lidocaine	Xylocaine, Octocaine, Lignospan, Alphacaine
Mepivacaine	Carbocaine, Polocaine, Scandonest
Prilocaine	Citanest
Phentolamine	OraVerse
Antibiotics	
Amoxicillin	Amoxil, Moxatag (ER)
Amoxicillin/clavulanic acid	Augmentin
Azithromycin	Tri-Pak, Z-Pak, Zithromax
Clindamycin	Cleocin
Doxycycline	Atridox, Doryx, Monodox, Periostat
Erythromycin	Ery-Tab, E.E.S
Metronidazole	Flagyl, Flagyl ER
Penicillin VK	Penicillin VK
Antifungals	
Clotrimazole	Mycelex
Fluconazole	Diflucan
Nystatin	Nilstat, Nystatin
Voriconazole	Vfend

Legend: ER - Extended Release formulation, **Inj** - Injectable solution, **sl** - Sublingual tablet or film, **Sol** - Oral solution

Table 3a. Most Common Prescribed Drugs in Dental Medicine

Generic	Brand Names
Antivirals	
Acyclovir	Zovirax, Sitavig (buccal tablets)
Penciclovir	Denavir
ValAcyclovir	Valtrex
Anxiolytics	
Diazepam	Valium
Triazolam	Halcion
Corticosteroids	
Dexamethasone	Decadron
Emergency Drugs	
Albuterol	Ventolin
Atropine	AtroPen (Inj)
Diphenydramine	Benadryl
Ephedrine	Akovaz (Inj)
Ephinephrine	EpiPen (Inj), Adrenalin, (Inj), Adrenaclick (Inj)
Flumazenil	Romazicon (Inj)
Hydrocortisone	Cortef
Lorazepam	Ativan
Naloxone	Narcan (Inj), Narcan (nasal spray)
Nitroglycerin	Nitrostat, NitroMist (oral spray)
Fluoride	
Fluoride tablets	Epiflur, Fluor-A-Day, Fluoritab, Ludent
Fluoride drops	Flura-drops, Luride drops, Pediaflor drops
Muscle Relaxants	
Baclofen	Lioresal, Gablofen (Inj)
Carisoprodol	Soma
Carisoprodol /aspirin/codeine	Soma compound with codeine
Cyclobenzaprine	Flexeril, Amrix (ER)
Metaxalone	Skelaxin
Orphenadrine	Norflex (Inj)
Tizanidine	Zanaflex
Salivary Management	
Cevimeline	Evoxac
Pilocarpine	Salagen
Glycopyrrolate	Cuvposa (Sol), Glycate
Tobacco Cessation	
Nicotine	Nicoderm (patch), Nicorette (gum), Nicotrol (nasal spray)
Bupropion	Zyban
Varenicline	Chantix

Legend: ER - Extended Release formulation, **Inj** - Injectable solution, **sl** - Sublingual tablet or film, **Sol** - Oral solution

Table 3b. Most Common Prescribed Drugs in 2017

Generic	Brand Names
Alprazolam	Xanax, Xanax ER
Amlodipine	Norvasc
Amoxicillin	Amoxil, Moxatag (ER)
Atorvastatin	Lipitor
Azithromycin	Tri-Pak, Z-Pak, Zithromax
Furosemide	Lasix
Gabapentin	Gralise, Horizant (ER), Neurontin
Hydrochlorothiazide	HCTZ, Microzide
Hydrocodone/APAP	Lortab, Norco, Vicodin
Ibuprofen	Motrin
Levothyroxine	Levothroid, Levoxyl, Synthroid, Unithroid
Lisinopril	Prinivil, Zestril
Losartan	Cozaar
Metformin	Fortamet (ER) Glucophage, Glumetza (ER), Riomet (Sol)
Metoprolol	Lopressor (Inj), Toprol
Omeprazole	Prilosec
Ondansetron	Zofran, Zuplenz (sl)
Prednisone	Deltasone, Prednisone
Sertraline	Zoloft
Zolpidem	Ambien, Edular (sl), Intermezzo, Zolpimist (oral spray)

Legend: ER - Extended Release formulation, **Inj** - Injectable solution, **sl** - Sublingual tablet or film, **Sol** - Oral solution

For generic-brand list: *https://www.rxlist.com/drugs/alpha_a.htm*
For drug pricings: *https://www.goodrx.com/drug-guide*